MEDICAL EXPERIMENTATION:
PERSONAL INTEGRITY AND SOCIAL POLICY

CLINICAL STUDIES

A North-Holland Frontiers Series

VOLUME 5

Edited by

A. G. BEARN
New York

D. A. K. BLACK
Manchester

H. H. HIATT
Boston

1974

NORTH-HOLLAND PUBLISHING COMPANY – AMSTERDAM · OXFORD
AMERICAN ELSEVIER PUBLISHING CO., INC. – NEW YORK

MEDICAL EXPERIMENTATION: PERSONAL INTEGRITY AND SOCIAL POLICY

CHARLES FRIED

Professor of Law, Law School of Harvard University,

Cambridge, Mass. 02138, U.S.A.

1974

NORTH-HOLLAND PUBLISHING COMPANY – AMSTERDAM · OXFORD
AMERICAN ELSEVIER PUBLISHING CO., INC. – NEW YORK

Library of Congress Catalog Card Number: 74 79334
ISBN North-Holland–series: 0 7204 7300 4
–volume: 0 7204 7305 5
ISBN American Elsevier – 0 444 10655 3

PUBLISHERS:
NORTH-HOLLAND PUBLISHING COMPANY – AMSTERDAM
NORTH-HOLLAND PUBLISHING COMPANY, LTD. – LONDON

SOLE DISTRIBUTORS FOR THE U.S.A. AND CANADA:
AMERICAN ELSEVIER PUBLISHING COMPANY, INC.
52 VANDERBILT AVENUE, NEW YORK, N.Y. 10017

PRINTED IN THE NETHERLANDS

for Howard Hiatt

Editors' preface

This series is complementary to the well-established 'Frontiers in Biology' series, edited by A. Neuberger and E. L. Tatum. The short general title 'Clinical Studies' does not fully indicate the purpose and scope of the series, which has indeed eluded our early efforts to find a title which would be both descriptive and comprehensive. There are two, somewhat separate, keynotes of the series—origin in medical departments, and clinical relevance. The series consists mainly of specially commissioned monographs, but does not exclude submitted manuscripts, or occasional reports of conferences on clearly defined topics. The main criteria of selection for the series are quality of material and presentation, in both of which we aim to achieve a high standard.

No sensible person would draw a rigid line in the bio-medical sciences between what is 'fundamental' and what is 'applied' or 'clinical'. In the same way, there are monographs in the 'Frontiers of Biology' series which have great clinical relevance; but in this series we hope to draw contributions from that area of scientific endeavour, often manifested in clinical academic departments which is concerned less with fundamental biology and more with problems arising in clinical medicine. We are well aware that modern medicine is firmly based on the fundamental sciences, including those which deal with behaviour; but we are equally conscious of the intensity and depth of the scientific work which is directly inspired by clinical problems. Some of this work consists of careful observation of nature's own experiments, but 'observation' now means something much more sophisticated than it did in the days of Auenbrugger and Laennec. The older techniques still have a place in studying the natural history of disease; but laboratory-based techniques have greatly extended the range of what can be observed. Partly because of this, and also because the fascination of clinical studies has always attracted keen minds, we see our editorial problem largely as one of critical selection, in view of the wide range of possible contributions to the series.

Contents

CHAPTER 1

Introduction

This essay, though long and in some respects perhaps exhaustive, does not seek to be definitive. There never will be a definitive treatment of the law and ethics of medical treatment in general, and so of medical experimentation in particular. Medicine is concerned with man's health, and human health is no more a fixed notion than is human nature with which it is directly correlated. It is neither surprising nor particularly unreasonable that in many cultures medicine is the province of religion. One need only recognize our own culture's inability successfully to integrate in or exclude from scientific medicine psychoanalytic theory and practice to see that each culture's definition of and approach to health implicates the widest range of philosophical presuppositions about man — both as an individual and as a social being. Even the view that medicine is concerned solely with the health of the body implies a view of the relation of body to person.

Medical experimentation, its proprieties and excesses, have been treated often and thoroughly in recent years.[1] The occasion

---

[1] J. Katz, *Experimentation with Human Beings* (1972) [hereinafter cited as Katz] is a massive and comprehensive collection of excerpts from materials bearing on all aspects of the subject. In addition it contains an extensive index. The work is invaluable for any serious researcher in the subject and I was greatly assisted by it. Two recent monographs of special interest are H. Beecher, *Research and the Individual — Human Studies* (1970) and P. Ramsey, *The Patient as Person* (1970). Finally two excellent recent symposia are vol. 98 *Daedalus — Journal of the American Academy of Arts & Sciences, Ethical Aspects of Experimentation with Human Subjects* (1969),

for yet another treatment, where there can be no definitive treatment, arises because these other treatments in pressing towards concrete conclusions, recognize but do not linger over those deepest, most difficult and most insoluble questions within which the particular subject is embedded. In this essay I shall reverse the usual, sensible impulse to trade philosophical and theoretical complexity for a modicum of usefulness. The exploration of philosophical, moral questions will hold center stage here, and concrete recommendations will be developed as by-products, hypotheses, tentative conclusions. There will be concrete conclusions and recommendations, but in the end it is the speculation and analysis which lead to them and which they illustrate that I offer as my particular contributions to this subject, a subject which most broadly is the relation of man to his body, the terms on which men care for each other, and the terms on which men and their bodies are at the disposal of the human groups of which they are a part.

The expanding capability of medicine and the recognition of an expanding responsibility to offer the best of care to everyone have forced a recognition of dilemmas that for centuries have been buried beneath the surface by common consent and professional reticence. Any thoughtful person now must know that if we do not engage in continuous and thorough medical experimentation we risk forgoing the benefits of new remedies, or poisoning ourselves with insufficiently tested new remedies, or indeed poisoning ourselves with accepted but unsound old remedies. Moreover, where we do not risk harm, we risk waste. And given our social commitment to make available to all what we offer to some, every expenditure is potentially multiplied a million fold, and in that perspective a useless therapy, a wasteful

---

also published as *Experimentation with Human Subjects* (P. Freund, ed. 1970) [hereinafter cited as *Daedalus*], and *New Dimensions in Legal and Ethical Concepts for Human Research*, 169 *Annals N. Y. Acad. Sci.* (1970) [hereinafter cited as *Annals*].

The most eloquent recent plea by a distinguished clinician and now a high official in the British National Health Service for experimentation and particularly for randomized clinical trials as part of a rational health policy is A. L. Cochrane, *Effectiveness and Efficiency* (1972).

procedure can cost the price of a year of schooling for the children of a whole region. As we make this commitment to equality, so too we commit ourselves to seeing these questions in terms of populations and generations, and in this perspective the individual, who was traditionally the unit of the physician's concern, becomes a fungible item in the mass, for otherwise it just is not possible to make the calculations and compute the costs.

It is in this perspective that the claims of experimentation have become so urgent. If medicine is to be viewed as caring for populations, then the information on which one acts becomes just one more factor to be prudently managed in developing an overall strategy for the best long-run discharge of this responsibility. Just as prudent calculations must be made regarding the comparative advantages of improved water supplies, better housing, inoculation programs and the like, so the costs of getting or not getting more information regarding new or old therapies must be weighed in the equation. And that is all there is to it.

But that is not all there is to it. The inhumanity and the professional arrogance of medical experimentation is one of the popular themes of western public discourse — at least since the Nuremberg trials. Many who have never even heard of the Nazi doctors see medical experimentation and the claims of the medical bureaucracy as yet another example of technocratic pretension, to be treated with suspicion and ultimately to be resisted. Doctors, drug companies and medical experimenters are subject to more searching publicity and to stricter controls than ever before in the name of the autonomy of the individual. Perhaps all this is a pointless flurry at the edges as politicians and journalists refuse to admit the inevitable. Or to the extent that the resistance is effective, perhaps it represents a harmful irrationality, wasting in the name of meaningless abstractions real resources that might be used to alleviate real misery.

Both tendencies are very powerful, nor do they have a unique bearing on medical experimentation. Similar conflicts are felt in the areas of criminal law, procedure and corrections, in the control of bureaucracies concerned with housing, education, employment, land use, the environment and technology. And though there are special interests that profit from the victories of one or the other side, the conflict is essentially one of ideas. In general those who favour an overall view in terms of groups and populations appear to have reason on their side. At any rate they have on their side what appears to be the apparatus of reason: statistics, calculations, predictions, cost-benefit analysis, linear programming, program budgeting and so on. On the other side are strong feeling, rhetoric, and often the conservative, stubborn force of the law. One of my major reasons for undertaking this study is to see if philosophical analysis, by deflating somewhat the pretensions of the first approach and rationalizing and clarifying the rhetoric of the second, cannot come up with something that is clear and coherent and at the same time true to our moral intuitions. This effort has been made before, at various levels of abstraction. It is an enterprise that began with Kant's attempt to develop a social, political, and personal morality that avoided what he called "the serpent-windings of utilitarianism". The most distinguished recent such work is John Rawls' *A Theory of Justice*. By taking medical experimentation as my subject, I hope to continue this effort, but focusing on a concrete application of theory and principles.

The Nazi doctors deliberately inflicted horrible suffering on helpless, unwilling subjects, just as distinguished doctors for generations before them deliberately infected unknowing poor, or ignorant, or retarded subjects with various diseases in order to study their progress and treatment. That kind of experimentation finds no defenders today. The issues today concern volunteers, paid or not, the use of children and incompetents who are also often "volunteered" by their guardians, and trials of new or old therapies on ill persons in the course of treating their very illness. It is the last kind of experimentation that will be the focus of this essay.

It is in this last category of experiment that the subtlest general questions are raised and the largest claims are made. These questions and claims will be used to focus the argumentation throughout the essay. Problems relating to children and incompetents I put aside. They are agonizingly difficult, but illuminate more the special status of infancy or incompetence than the questions of experimentation.

In the category I am interested in varying modalities of a new but promising treatment will be tried on an ill person, in part to cure him and in part to evaluate and perfect the new treatment. Often traditional alternatives are ineffective or have serious drawbacks. Thus, it is said, an effort is being made not only to cure the individual patient but also to help others similarly afflicted. The most sophisticated and presently most fashionable version of this form of therapeutic investigation is the randomized clinical trial (RCT), in which the allocation of a patient to a particular treatment category or its alternative — sometimes an alternative therapy, sometimes a placebo, that is no therapy at all — is done at random. In this way if there are enough cases the influence of extraneous factors on the outcome can be washed out and the effects attributable to the treatment under investigation isolated. A further refinement is double-blind or single-blind trials in which the results of the random assignment are kept from the subject and/or the investigators until after the completion of the trial. The RCT has many points of appeal to medical researchers. Since the factors influencing health and illness are so numerous, a satisfactory theoretical demonstration of the full causal efficacy of a therapy is hard to come by. And for the same reason comparative studies, regression analyses and the like might fail to notice the significance of some interfering factor. Finally, in a field fraught with professional rivalries and vested interests, it is often only the statistically most impregnable demonstrations that will convince the skeptics.

Complementing the statistical allure of the RCT is its appeal to what many think is the most rational conception of medical care for populations as a whole. The RCT invites us to look at diseases as afflicting populations and at therapies as reducing the incidence of disease. The RCT by leading not to accounts of a few successful cures but to comparisons of mortality or morbidity

rates in large groups asks the questions that many think are the
relevant ones. Nor on this view does the individual have anything
to complain about. Ideally randomization will not be resorted
to unless and until there is a real division of opinion regarding
the relative merits of the two therapies (including on occasion
placebo therapy), so that no one is being deprived *ex ante* of the
"better" therapy. Moreover, anyone who is a patient in a system
that regularly has recourse to RCT testing has overall a better
chance of being treated with more effective therapies at less cost.
In any case, what else is to be done if new treatments are to be
developed, the sum total of misery lessened? Somehow the new
must be evaluated against the old if progress is to be made, and
often the RCT is the best way of accomplishing this.

Because the RCT expresses so neatly a particular way of looking
at the ends of medicine, at social policy in general and at the
rights and obligations of individuals implicated in the implementation of the policy, I shall make the RCT the particular
concern of this essay. In examining the claims made for the RCT,
objections to it, in considering qualifications and proposing
acceptable modalities and alternatives to the RCT I hope to
clarify to some extent the widening circle of issues related to it:
The conflict between care for individuals and care for groups, the
proper ends of medicine, the significance of consent and the
meaning of full disclosure in preserving individual autonomy, the
contrast between fairness and efficiency in social schemes, and the
function of compensation to effect fairness after the fact.

I shall begin in the next chapter with a review of the principal
legal doctrines bearing on the rights and liabilities, permissions
and prohibitions relating to those acting and acted upon in
medical research. In this way we can establish some basic conceptual distinctions, identify the issues that have attracted sufficient social attention to be dealt with in legal doctrine, and put
a concrete foundation under our ethical speculations. It is striking
that much of what concerns us has not been dealt with directly
in court decisions or legal codes, although some quasi-legal
sources like the Nuremberg Code and the Declaration of Helsinki

and some administrative materials like the Department of Health, Education and Welfare *Policy on Protection of Human Subjects*[2] come closer. In the end, to determine the law regarding RCT's we will have to rely to a great extent on extrapolation from existing precedents and general doctrine. Such extrapolation, however convincing, is an uncertain guide to what the first actual case will hold. For in seeing what the implications of a precedent or doctrine are a court may decide to abandon or modify it. And this is just one reason why even the most definitive statement of the existing law is only a first step: not only can the law change, but it is our responsibility to judge if the law is wise, and if it is not wise to urge that it be changed and to show what the changes should be. This is what the succeeding chapters seek to do. Chapters 3 and 4 argue that personal care is both an interest and a right, and in the course of that argument develop a notion of rights at variance with much economic writing in the health care field. Chapter 5 asks how the theoretical notions in the prior chapters and especially the rights in personal care come together to form a coherent whole, given the demands of responsibility for patients not only on a one-by-one basis but as members of social groups and populations. The method is to confront the theoretical notions of the previous discussion with the realities of medical economics and medical practice. The final chapter applies the more general ideas and arguments to the issues of medical experimentation in order to test them, deepen them, and bring them down to earth in concrete recommendations.

---

[2] *Federal Register*, vol. 38, no. 194, October 9, 1973, page 27882. The proposed rules are substantially similar to the earlier *NIH Guide* published in 1971.

The legal context of
medical experimentation

This chapter presents the principles of American law applicable to medical experimentation. Since, as Tocqueville remarked, in the United States grave public questions tend to be seen as legal questions, such a presentation should go beyond parochial concerns and introduce as well in a concrete and practical way the issues and concepts to be confronted more theoretically in subsequent chapters.

The principal category defining rights and duties in medical practice are found in the law of torts. Although the professional relationship is one of a contract of services, for reasons that will readily appear contractual notions are not prominent in this area. So also the criminal law is concerned with some of the wrongs that in a civil suit would appear as battery or negligence. However, little need be said about criminal liability, since criminal prosecutions are rarely brought, and in any case the applicable concepts of the criminal law are the same as those of the civil law, except they are far more sparingly and stringently applied. Finally, we will have to consider a number of administrative regulations which are highly influential in controlling and defining standards for the conduct of medical experimentation.

2.1. General principles

If we seek the legal principles governing the relation of medical practitioners to their subjects, we must with few exceptions look to the law of battery or negligence.[1] Both these causes of action are tort actions brought by or on behalf of a plaintiff who believes that he has been legally and/or factually injured and is seeking legal redress in the form of substantial monetary damages. In most general terms a battery is committed when there is an intentional contact with the plaintiff's body, and that contact neither has been consented to nor is legally privileged.[2] The tort of negligence is committed when a legally protected interest of the plaintiff is invaded as a result of conduct on the part of the defendant which falls below the standard of care reasonably to be expected from ordinary members of the community, or if the defendant has some special skill or knowledge, from persons possessing such special qualifications.[3] Some suits in which persons vindicate their rights against doctors or hospitals involve conduct to which the plaintiff has not consented[4] — or because of in-

---

[1] See generally W. Prosser, *Torts* 34–37, 102–07, 161–66 (4th ed. 1971). Two principal treatises on medical practice are D. Louisell and H. Williams, *Medical Malpractice* (1970, Suppl. 1972) and *Medical Malpractice* (D. McDonald, ed. 1971). The general setting is supplied by Jaffe, "Law as a System of Control," and Freund, "Legal Frameworks for Human Experimentation," both in *Daedalus* (1969). This symposium on medical experimentation [hereinafter cited as *Daedalus*] also appeared as a separate volume, *Experimentation with Human Subjects* (P. Freund, ed. 1970).

Numerous Articles and Comments have appeared on the law of experimentation. See, e.g., Note 75, *Harv. L. Rev.* 1445 (1962); Note, "Experimentation," 46 *Neb. L. Rev.* 87 (1967); Note, "Experimentation on Human Beings," 20 *Stan. L. Rev.* 99 (1967); Comment, "Non-Therapeutic Research Involving Human Subjects," 24 *Syr. L. Rev.* 1067 (1973). For a full bibliography, see J. Katz, *Experimentation with Human Beings* (1972).

[2] See *Restatement (Second) of Torts* § 13 (1965), [hereinafter cited as *ALI*]; and Prosser, supra ch. 2 § 9.

[3] See *ALI* § 281–96; Prosser, supra ch. 5.

[4] E.g. Rogers v. Lumbermens Mut. Cas. Co., 119 So. 2d 649 (La. Cir. Ct. App. 1960); Mohr v. Williams, 95 Minn. 261, 104 N.W. 12 (1905); see, e.g., Plante, "An Analysis of Informed Consent," 36 *Ford. L. Rev.* 639 (1968); Waltz and Schennman, "Informed Consent to Therapy," 64 *Nw. U. L. Rev.* 628 (1970).

complete disclosures has not validly consented[5] — and thus constitute a battery upon the plaintiff; or they charge that the practitioner has performed the actions to which the plaintiff has in fact consented without the exercise of customary care, that is negligently.

The central concept of battery is the offense to personal dignity which occurs when another impinges on one's bodily integrity without full and valid consent. A punch in the stomach or being doused with a pail of water are classic examples. It is not necessary to show that one has been physically injured, much less that one has suffered financial loss. The injury is to dignity.[6] That being the case, law suits have been brought and won against doctors who performed needed and successful operations, but without the consent of their patients.[7] In negligence, by contrast, it is necessary to prove substantial injuries, preferably with pecuniary implications.[8] A tendency has arisen, however, to designate actions against doctors as "malpractice" irrespective of which of these two distinct theories is the basis of the action. The term malpractice is in truth no more than an index heading under which causes of action against doctors are collected. Treating the case, for instance, in which a physician obtains consent to a hysterectomy by misleading or incomplete disclosures, simply as a case of malpractice might lead to serious confusion. That the doctor failed to get proper consent from his patient may have been negligent;[9] but the unconsented to operation is itself a battery. And if the suit is governed by the legal principles of negligence, it might well be open to the doctor to argue that

---

[5] See supra note 4 and authorities cited in Comment, 24 *Syr. L. Rev.* 1067, supra note 1 at nn. 37–39.

[6] See *ALI* and Prosser, supra note 1.

[7] E.g. Mohr v. Williams, 95 Minn. 261, 104 N.W. 12 (1905). For a parallel case in a trespass to land, see Longenecker v. Zimmerman, 175 Kan. 719, 267 P. 2d. 543 (1954) (defendant had plaintiff's trees treated erroneously believing them to be her own).

[8] See Prosser, supra note 1, at 143–44.

[9] See, e.g., Wilson v. Scott, 412 S.W. 2d 299 (Tex. 1967); cf. Davis v. Wyeth Laboratories, Inc., 399 F. 2d 121 (9th Cir. 1968).

whatever the patient may have believed, the fact of the matter is that far from having been injured by the operation she was substantially benefited. This argument would be unavailable in a battery action, because the plaintiff is complaining about the indignity involved in having one's body significantly "intermeddled with" (as the lawyers say) without having had the opportunity intelligently to decide whether to consent to such a procedure.

Whether it is desirable to elide the distinction between the two doctrines, assimilating both to the principles of negligence is a question which might be said to include the whole subject of this essay. For it is the law of battery which vindicates in a rather uncompromising way the principle of physical integrity of the individual,[10] an integrity which is violated not only by forceful interference, but by interference where consent was procured through deceptive or incomplete disclosures. The law of negligence, by contrast, speaking as it does in terms of "reasonableness" and "substantial harm", invites inquiry from the very outset into questions of balance, questions of the social utility of what the medical practitioner did, questions of the practitioner's conformance to community practice, and finally questions of the substantiality of the plaintiff's harm. By moving from battery to negligence via the hybrid rubric of malpractice, one is moving from a standard which recognizes a right in the individual to a standard which sees the law as a forum for weighing and determining controverted questions of relative social utility.

In general, one acts negligently in failing to abide by the standard of due care. The concept of due care is compounded of two elements. First, in requiring that a person act reasonably the law invites an inquiry into the purposes of his action. If an actor's goal is sufficiently important and urgent, then he may be justified in imposing a corresponding level of risk on those who are in his way.[11] Second, due care refers also to the way in which the (let

---

[10] See Freund, in *Daedalus*, supra note 1.

[11] United States v. Carroll Towing Co., 159 F. 2d 169 (2d Cir. 1947); Noll v. Marian, 347 Pa. 213, 32 A. 2d. 18 (1943); and see generally C. Fried, *An Anatomy of Values* (1970).

us assume) proper goal is pursued. It may be quite proper to exceed the speed limit when driving an ill person to the hospital for emergency treatment, but one is still obliged to use due care as one drives, by keeping a lookout, sounding the horn and so on.[12]

The usual case in which a doctor is sued for negligence by his patient involves a charge of lack of due care of the latter sort. The standard of due care is that degree of care and prudence exercised by reasonable men in the community. This notion, obviously, needs qualification or specification if it is to be applied to medical practitioners, since ordinary reasonable men in the community do not engage in the practice of medicine. And, if a person has special knowledge or a special skill he will be held to the care exercised generally by those with that skill or knowledge.[13] Since a medical practitioner holds himself out as having certain skills, the law judges him accordingly, whether he has them or not.[14]

There is a sense, however, in which the law is more lenient towards doctors, for it remits the question of what is due care in medicine to the medical profession itself. In order to prevail in a negligence suit against the doctor, the plaintiff must prove not that what the defendant did was unreasonable, but that there is no accepted body of medical opinion according to which what the defendant did might be judged reasonable.[15] Neither judge nor jury is entitled to determine that the practice of an accepted "school" of medicine is itself unreasonably lax.[16]

This deference to the medical profession in determining what is reasonableness in medicine is, perhaps, appropriate where what

---

[12] See, e.g., La Marra v. Adam, 164 Pa. Super 268, 63 A. 2d 497 (1949).

[13] *ALI* § 289; Prosser, supra note 1, at 161–66.

[14] In this sense the law of negligence and that of contracts coalesce; one might either say that a surgeon is negligent in undertaking to treat someone if he does not exercise the usual levels of skill, or one might say that a surgeon implicitly warrants in the sense of making a contractual promise that he will exercise at least the ordinary level of skill in undertaking to treat a patient. Either way, it is by the higher standards that the reasonableness of the care exercised is judged. This is why I have said at the outset that doctrines of contract law are not especially applicable to our concerns. See Prosser, supra note 1, at 162–63.

[15] See Wiggins v. Piver, 276 N.C. 134, 171 S.E. 2d 393 (1970).

[16] See Prosser, supra note 1, at 163.

is in question relates to the proper execution of this or that medical procedure. Where, however, this deference is paid to the profession in respect to standards of disclosure and consent as well,[17] then the law has to my mind wrongly abjured its own responsibilities. For the question of when a patient, a layman has put himself into the hands of doctors, when he has submitted himself to the judgements of the profession by giving his consent should be a question not for the medical profession but for the general community from which this layman comes. It may well be that some respected practitioners will not tell patients of certain risks in some proposed therapy believing the information to be irrelevant.[18] But whether this is a proper judgement is no longer only a medical question; rather it is a question to be arbitrated between doctors on the one hand and layman on the other. It is perhaps a further consequence of the occasional blurring of the conceptual distinction between negligence and battery within the all inclusive term of malpractice, that the standards and forms of proof appropriate to negligence are improperly imported into the quite different question of whether a patient has validly consented to a particular procedure.[19] This issue brings us, then, to a more detailed consideration of the meaning and function of the concept of consent in the law relating to medical practice.

2.2. *Consent*

The major premise justifying intentional invasions of an individual's bodily integrity is consent.[20] Reasonableness, social utility,

[17] See, e.g., Di Filippo v. Preston, 53 Del. 539, 173 A. 2d 333 (1961); Kennedy v. Parrott, 243 N.C. 355, 90 S.E. 2d 754 (1956); Wilson v. Scott, 412 S.W. 2d 299 (Tex. 1967); *Syr. L. Rev.* supra note 1, at n. 38.

[18] See, e.g., Manen v. Ellsworth, 3 Wash, App. 298, 474 P. 2d 909 (1970) (risk of perforation during esophagoscope examination); Kaplan v. Haines, 96 N.J. Super 242, 232 A. 2d 840 (1967), aff'd 51 N.J. 404, 241 A. 2d 235 (1968); Wilson v. Scott, supra.

[19] Wilson v. Scott, supra note 17.

[20] My position is supported by the decisions in Canterbury v. Spence, 464 F. 2d

the impinging actor's high purposes, are all relevant where the actor is pursuing some other goal and the impingement on a person's body is an accidental or unavoidable concomitant of that pursuit. But where, as in medical practice and medical experimentation, that impingement just *is* the purpose of the conduct, then—with a very few exceptions—consent is needed to justify it.

2.2.1. The meaning of consent

The consent which justifies what the law calls "intermeddling" with a person's body is free and informed consent. To be effective the consent must be to the particular contact with the person in question, and if procured by "fraud or mistake as to the essential character" of the conduct it is invalid.[21] Thus a husband has been held guilty of battery where he had intercourse with his wife without informing her that he was infected with a veneral disease.[22] Consent to treatment has been held to be ineffective in cases where the defendant has falsely represented himself to be a qualified doctor.[23]

And it is not just active fraud or concealment which destroys consent. The doctor who obtains consent has the duty to give the facts the patient needs to make an informed choice.[24] He must give the patient his diagnosis of the illness and its prognosis without treatment. He must tell the patient about the benefits and risks of the treatment, and how likely they are. And some courts

772 (D.C. Cir. 1972); Wilkinson v. Vesey, 295 A. 2d 676 (R.I. 1972); Cooper v. Roberts, 220 Pa. Super. 260, 286 A. 2d 647 (1971). *ALI* § 49; Prosser, supra note 1, at 101.

[21] *ALI* § 55.

[22] E.g. Crowell v. Crowell, 180 N.C. 516, 105 S.E. 206 (1920), reh'g denied, 18 N.C. 66, 106 S.E. 149 (1921); DeVall v. Strunk, 96 S.W. 2d 245 (Tex. Civ. App. 1936); State v. Lankford, 29 Del. 594, 102 A. 63 (1917).

[23] See, e.g., Bartell v. State, 106 Wis. 342, 82 N.W. 142 (1900).

[24] In addition to the authorities in notes 1, 22 and 23 supra, see Notes, 55 *Calif. L. Rev.* 1396 (1967); 71 *Dick. L. Rev.* 675 (1967); 4 *Duquesne L. Rev.* 450 (1966); 17 *U.C.L.A. L. Rev.* 758 (1970); 79 *Yale L. J.* 1533 (1970).

For recent cases, see Canterbury v. Spence, 464 F. 2d 772 (D.C. Cir 1972); Salgo v. Stanford U. B'd. of Trustees, 154 Cal. App. 2d 560, 317 P. 2d 170 (1957).

have said that the patient must also be told about the hazards and advantages of alternative forms of treatment.[25]

2.2.2. *Qualifications of the requirement of informed consent*

The law requires disclosure only of *material* facts, so that the failure to disclose some exceedingly remote risk is consistent with valid consent barring the patient's battery suit against the doctor.[26] A recent decision has reasoned, however, that even a one in a million chance of contracting polio — in connection with live virus immunization — was a material hazard requiring disclosure, given the seriousness of the consequences and the equally remote risk of the adult patient in fact contracting polio without vaccination.[27] Further, if a person gives the reasonable appearance of consenting, then that is as good as actual consent.[28] Similarly, where a patient is unconscious, the courts have held that a doctor may assume that the patient would have consented to emergency or other treatment that most reasonable people under the circumstances would have desired.[29]

These qualifications of the requirement of consent have been argued to show that the requirement is not itself an absolute and that like everything else it too must yield to claims of the greater good of the greater number.[30] Where a patient is being operated upon for an appendectomy and the surgeon discovers ovarian cysts, to sew that patient up, seek consent, and then reoperate for the cysts would be to expose to the inconvenience and risks of a second operation the vast majority of women who would consent,

---

[25] Canterbury v. Spence, supra; Durham v. Wright, 423 F. 2d 940 (3rd. Cir. 1970); Campbell v. Oliva, 424 F. 2d 1244 (6th Cir. 1970).

[26] See supra note 24. It should be noted that the decisions cited in note 24 make clear that relevance is to be judged in terms of what the patient reasonably would need to know to make a sound decision.

[27] Davis V. Wyeth Laboratories, Inc., 399 F. 2d 121 (9th Cir. 1968). The case was a suit against the manufacturer of the vaccine, not the administering medical personnel.

[28] O'Brien v. Cunard Steamship Co., 154 Mass. 272, 28 N.E. 266 (1891).

[29] Kennedy v. Parrott, supra note 17.

[30] Jaffe, supra note 1.

for the sake of a small minority with aberrant views.[31] However, nothing in these cases justifies going ahead where there is knowledge or reason to believe that the particular patient would *not* consent to a procedure.[32] These doctrines of apparent, implied or presumed consent, on the contrary, all accept the premise that medical intervention requires consent. Their only qualification of that doctrine is to allow the intervention without *explicit* consent, which is quite different from overriding a patient's wishes, where those wishes are known.

The so-called therapeutic privilege presents another, rather different qualification of the general requirement for full and informed consent. This doctrine justifies a doctor in withholding information from his patient, if he reasonably believes that disclosing it would not be in the patient's interest, that it would interfere with the best treatment of the patient.[33] Thus it might be justifiable not to tell a patient that he is suffering from, say, cancer, and to treat him without obtaining a consent informed by knowledge of the diagnosis and prospects.[34] Similarly, courts have held that a doctor may fail to disclose certain risks inherent in a therapy he is proposing to the patient, if being told of these risks would unduly disturb the patient and interfere with his cure.[35] There

---

[31] E.g., Kennedy v. Parrott, supra note 17.

[32] Compare Clayton v. New Dreamland Roller Skating Rink, Inc., 14 N.J. Super, 390, 82 A. 2d 458 (1951) (battery to attempt to set arm over plaintiff's protest); Corn v. French, 71 Nev. 280, 289 P. 2d 173 (1955) (patient signed consent form referring to mastectomy, but had specifically told surgeon she did not want her breast removed); In re Brook's Estate, 32 Ill 2d 361, 205 N.E. 2d 435 (1965) (Jehovah's Witness had right to refuse blood transfusion); contra, Application of President and Directors of Georgetown College, Inc., 331 F. 2d 100 (1964) (treatment authorized in spite of refusal by adult patient). See generally, Cantor, "A Patient's Decision to Decline Life-Saving Medical Treatment: Bodily Integrity versus the Preservation of Life," 26 *Rutgers L. Rev.* 228 (1973).

[33] See Canterbury v. Spence, supra note 24, at 789; Salgo v. Stanford U. B'd. of Trustees, supra note 24, at 578, 181.

[34] Cf. Curran, "Governmental Regulation of the Use of Human Subjects in Medical Research: The Approach of Two Federal Agencies," *Daedalus* 542.

[35] See Patrick v. Sedwick, 391 P. 2d 453 (Alaska 1964); DiFilippo v. Preston, 53 Del. 539, 173 A. 2d 333 (Sup. Ct. 1961); Natanson v. Kline, 186 Kan. 393, 350 P. 2d 1093 (1960), on reh'g, 187 Kan. 186, 354 P. 2d 670 (1960).

has been a great deal of loose talk of this "therapeutic privilege",
leading to the impression that just referring to the privilege a doctor
is justified in ignoring the obligation fully to inform his patient, if
only he believes he is acting in that patient's best interest. The
privilege and the arguments for it in no way support this loose
view.

First, the doctor who has made less than full disclosure must
justify his therapy in terms of the particular patient's interests.[36]
There is nothing in the authorities establishing this privilege
which would allow the doctor to rely on the interests of others,
social interests, general inconvenience or the like. *Second*, the
claim the doctor must make is that the information would itself
lead to serious distress interfering with a cure. It would be a
complete perversion of this notion to argue that a doctor is
justified in withholding information because a patient would,
quite calmly, on the basis of that information withhold his consent from a therapy which the doctor judged desirable.[37] Thus,
the therapeutic privilege is a qualification of the doctor's obligation to obtain consent only in so far as it may be assumed that
the patient would, if he were in a position to judge, ratify the
doctor's decision. If the information is withheld just in order to
subvert what the patient would choose if he had the information,
then the privilege itself is abused and the authorities establishing
it do not support such abuse.

2.2.3. Overriding the patient's failure to consent

There are a number of situations in which doctors are justified
in proceeding without consent, even when they know that if they

---

[36] Bonner v. Moran, 126 F. 2d 121 (D.C. Cir. 1941); Masden v. Harrison, Muskey
v. Harrison, Foster v. Harrison (unreported Mass. Sup. Jud. Ct) discussed in Curran, "A Problem of Consent, Kidney Transplantation in Minors," 34 *N.Y.U.L.
Rev.* 891 (1959); and in 24 *Syr. L. Rev.* 1067, at nn. 52–54 and accompanying text
(1973); but cf. Freund, "Introduction" to *Daedalus* at xvi (when uniquely suited to
experiment and no discernible hazard).

[37] ". . . the privilege does not accept the paternalistic notion that the physician
may remain silent simply because divulgence might prompt the patient to forego

sought consent it would not be given. Children, insane persons, and other incompetents may be treated in the name of their own best interests, and in spite of their avowed wishes and preferences.[38] This is because the law judges that persons in those categories are unable to make rational decisions regarding their welfare. As I have indicated in the Introduction, I am leaving out of account in this essay the special problems of these groups. It might be mentioned in passing, however, that the tendency of the law has been to limit greatly what may be done to children and incompetents just because they are unable to give effective consent. And those who act for them are strictly charged to act only in the manifest interests of those persons. They may not, for instance, volunteer them for experimentation which will not directly benefit them, or for organ donations and the like.[39]

Finally, doctors have been allowed to override the expressed wishes of their patients where the treatment they sought to impose was intended to protect not the patient but a third party or the public in general. Thus it has been held that persons may be compelled to receive vaccinations;[40] and the compelled quarantine of persons with contagious diseases has been permitted.[41] Nothing has justified, however, going further and compelling a person to confer a benefit against his will, for instance by ordering him to donate an organ or blood of a rare type.[42] Thus, in the case of experimentation, failure to abide by the requirements of fully informed consent could not be justified in accordance with these doctrines, since the subject who refuses to submit to experimentation does not by his refusal constitute a danger to others; he merely refuses to confer a benefit. One might, of course,

---

therapy the physician feels the patient really needs...." Canterbury v. Spence, 464, F. 2d 772, 789 (D.C. Cir. 1972).

[38] See supra note 32.

[39] Ibid.

[40] Jacobson v. Massachusetts, 197 U.S. 11 (1904).

[41] See, e.g., McGuire v. Amyx, 317 Mo. 1061, 297 S.W. 968 (1927) and annotation in 54 *A.L.R.* 644.

[42] See supra note 36, and Fried, supra note 11, at 200–206.

question whether this distinction is a rational or useful one. It is quite clear that it is one that the law makes.

2.2.4. *Withdrawal of consent and the continuing duty to disclose*

Although there are far fewer cases dealing with this matter, the doctrine appears to be well established that consent at least to an interference with bodily integrity may be withdrawn at any time. The fact that the consenting person had previously promised or even contracted not to withdraw his consent has never been found to bind him, should he later wish to change his mind.[43] Some balancing of convenience may be allowed where making one person's withdrawal effective requires affirmative action by another,[44] but this would not justify further positive impositions after a desire to withdraw has been expressed. For this reason it would certainly not be proper to continue treating a person after he has withdrawn his consent to that treatment, even though honoring his withdrawal might seriously inconvenience the further conduct of some experiment.

Since the obligation to make full disclosure and to obtain effective consent is well established, and the right to withdraw consent — though infrequently discussed — is also established beyond question, the issue naturally arises whether there is not a duty on the part of the physician to make periodic disclosures of fresh information, so that the patient might intelligently decide whether or not to withdraw his consent. The physician's initial disclosure, together with his acting upon the resulting consent would be sufficient to create a continuing duty to act affirmatively, and thus to make relevant disclosures from time to time. In particular, a doctor, who has undertaken treatment, has the duty to disclose that the treatment is not working and that better or in

---

[43] See State v. Williams, 75 N.C. 134 (1876); *ALI* § 254; Freund, supra note 1; *USDHEW, NIH, Institutional Guide to DHEW Policy on Protection of Human Subjects* (1971) [hereinafter cited as *NIH*] (Guide specifically requires that the subject be informed that he may withdraw consent at any time).

[44] See Heard v. Weardale [1915] A.C. 67 (House of Lords).

any case alternative treatment would be available elsewhere.[45] The only argument that would qualify this duty relates to the burden and inconvenience that might be involved in continually coming back to the patient with fresh disclosures.[46]

2.3. General legal principles applied to medical experimentation[47]

At the outset we must distinguish between therapeutic and non-therapeutic experimentation.[48] Experimentation is clearly non-therapeutic when it is carried out on a person solely to obtain information of use to others, and in no way to treat some illness that the experimental subject might have. Experimentation is therapeutic when a therapy is tried with the sole view of determining the best way of treating that patient. There is a sense, as a number of commentators have observed, in which so far as there is more or less uncertainty about the best way to proceed in the patient's case, treatment is often experimental.[49] Also what is learned in

---

[45] See Chalmers et al., "Controlled Studies in Clinical Cancer Research," 287 *N. Engl. J. Med.* 75 (July 13, 1972).

[46] See Baldor v. Rogers, 81 So. 2d 658, 662, 55 A.L.R. 2d 453 (Fla. 1955); Tvedt v. Havgen, 70 N.D. 338, 294 N.W. 183 (1940); Dietze v. King, 184 F. Supp. 944, 949 (E.D.Va. 1960).

[47] See generally Katz, supra note 1; Berger, "Reflections on Law and Experimental Medicine," 15 *U.C.L.A. L. Rev.* 436 (1968); Freund, supra note 1; Freund, "Ethical Problems in Human Experimentation," 273 *N. Eng. J. Med.* 687 (1965). Hirsh, "The Medico-Legal Framework for Medical Research" in *New Dimensions in Legal and Ethical Concepts for Human Research*, 169 Annals N.Y. Acad. Sci. (1970) [hereinafter cited as *Annals*]; Jaffe, supranote 1; Kaplan, "Experimentation — An Articulation of a New Myth," 46 *Neb. L. Rev.* 87 (1967); Note, 75 *Harv. L. Rev.* 1445 (1962); Note, 20 *Stan. L. Rev.* 99 (1967); Note, *Syr. L. Rev.* 1067 (1973).

[48] See Halushka v. University of Saskatchewan, 53 D.L.R. 2d 436 (1965); Hyman v. Jewish Chronic Disease Hosp., 42 Misc. 2d 427, 248 N.Y.S. 2d 245 (Sup. Ct. 1964); rev'd per curiam, 21 App. Div. 2d 495, 251 N.Y.S. 2d 818, rev'd 15 N.Y. 2d 317, 206 N.E. 2d 338, 258 N.Y.S. 2d 397 (1965); *NIH, Guide*; Capron, "The Law of Genetic Therapy," in Katz, supra note 1, at 574; Grad, "Regulation of Clinical Research by the State," in *Annals*; "Syposium," 36 *Fordham L. Rev.* 673 (1968).

[49] See Fortner v. Koch, 272 Mich. 273, 261 N.W. 762 (1835); Freund, supra note 1; Grad, supra; Katz, supra.

treating one patient will be of use in treating others. This may
be so, but it in no way obscures the distinction between therapeutic and non-therapeutic research, since therapeutic research is
carried out only and only so far as that subject's interests require.
Any benefits to others are incidental to this dominant goal. These
are the clear cases at the extreme.

There are in practice large numbers of gradations in between.
Much research is mainly therapeutic, in the sense that the patients'
interests are foremost, but nevertheless things may be done which
are not dictated solely by the need to treat that patient: tests
may be continued even after all the information needed to determine the best treatment of the particular patient have already
been completed; or substances may be injected for a period or
in doses not strictly necessary for the cure of that patient, but with
the motive of developing information of use to others.[50] Moving
in from the clear case at the other extreme, that of non-therapeutic
research, it must be recognized that persons who become research
subjects in non-therapeutic experimentation may often be the
beneficiaries of a degree of medical attention which they might
not otherwise enjoy, and which thus redounds to their benefit.[51]
And there are all possible degrees and gradations in between.

2.3.1. Non-therapeutic experimentation[52]

No special doctrines apply to non-therapeutic experimentation.
Indeed, to the extent that the experimentation is non-therapeutic,
the fact that it is being carried out by doctors should be entirely
irrelevant. The usual privileges under which doctors work, and
the usual special doctrines according to which the liabilities of
doctors are judged should not be applicable, since they proceed
from the premise that the doctor must be given considerable
latitude as he works in the presumed interests of his patient.

---

[50] See *NIH*, at 6.

[51] This was argued in defense of the experiments in Hyman v. Jewish Chronic
Disease Hospital discussed in Katz, supra, chapter 1.

[52] See authorities cited supra note 47.

But that is not the case in non-therapeutic research. The doctor confronts his subject simply as a scientist.

In general, the law imposes a strict duty of disclosure, wherever an individual with a great deal to lose is exposed to a risk or is asked to relinquish rights by someone with considerably greater knowledge.[53] And this is true, whether the relation is one of buyer and seller or involves some public interest. Persons selling cosmetics,[54] automobiles[55] or pharmaceuticals[56] are required to make full disclosures of all the hazards involved in the products they sell. But policemen seeking damaging admissions from suspects are also required to issue a warning of constitutional rights and to offer legal assistance before those rights are waived.[57] There is no reason why the case should be any different where a researcher asks an experimental subject to risk his health.

Indeed the case might be made that the developing doctrines of strict liability would argue for the imposition of liability without fault, and regardless of disclosures for harm occasioned in the course of non-therapeutic experimentation.[58] In general, it is

[53] See generally Prosser, supra note 1, at § 99; Calabresi, "Toward a Test for Strict Liability in Torts," 81 *Yale L. J.*, 1055 (1972).

[54] Larsen v. General Motors Corp., 391 F. 2d 495 (8th Cir. 1968); Witt v. Chrysler Corp., 15 Mich. App. 576, 167 N.W. 2d 100 (1969), Blitzstein v. Ford Motor Co., 288 F. 2d 738 (5th Cir. 1961).

[55] Crotty v. Shartenberg's-New Haven, Inc., 147 Conn. 460, 162 A. 2d 513 (1960) (hair remover); Reynolds v. Sun Ray Drug Company, 135 N.J.L. 475, 52 A. 2d 666 (Ct. Err. & App. 1947) (lipstick); Esborg v. Bailey Drug Co., 61 Wash. 2d 347, 378 P. 2d 298 (1963) (hair tint).

[56] Martin v. Bengue, Inc., 25 N.J. 359, 136 A. 2d 626 (1957); Marcus v. Specific Pharmaceuticals, 82 N.Y.S. 2d 194 (N.Y. Sup. Ct. 1948); Halloran v. Parke, Davis & Co., 245 App. Div. 727, 280 N.Y.S. 58 (1935).

[57] Miranda v. Arizona, 384 U.S. 436 (1966).

[58] See Calabresi, "Reflections on Medical Experimentation" in *Daedalus*; Freund, in *Daedalus*; Havighurst, "Compensating Persons Injured in Human Experimentation" 169 *Science* 153 (1970); Note, "Medical Experimentation Insurance" 70 *Colum. L. Rev.* 965 (1970); cf. Ehrenzweig" Compulsory Hospital-Accident Insurance: A Needed First Step Toward the Displacement of Liability for Medical Malpractice" 31 *U. Chi. L. Rev.* 279 (1964); R. Keeton, "Compensation for Medical Accidents" 121 *U. Pa. L. Rev.* 590 (1973); Note, "Medical Malpractice Litigation: Some Suggested Improvements and a Possible Alternative" 18 *U. Fla. L. Rev.* 623 (1966).

coming to be believed that those who are in a better position to appreciate the risks of a course of conduct, who are in a better position to insure against those risks or otherwise spread their cost to the broadest group of beneficiaries, and finally whose responsible decisions in evaluating the propriety of the risks we can influence by imposing upon them the costs of those decisions, should be strictly liable (that is liable without fault) for the risks that their conduct imposes.[59] These conditions are amply met in the case of non-therapeutic experimentation. Finally, if the financial pressures of caring for and compensating subjects injured in non-therapeutic experiments meant that experimenters exercised greater caution and carefully evaluated the benefits to be expected from the research, this would be a highly desirable consequence. It is for this reason that a number of commentators have suggested either strict liability for non-therapeutic experimentation or some form of compulsory medical experimentation insurance. In either case the experimental subject would be assured of proper medical care as well as compensatory payments for any injuries he suffers in the experiment. Since most subjects of non-therapeutic experimentation are either idealistic persons for whom the small amounts of compensation are not a significant inducement, or disadvantaged persons for whom the small compensation acts as an all too significant inducement, this added responsibility would seem fair and appropriate.

2.3.2. Therapeutic experimentation

Legal decisions and commentators have always stated that a practitioner is only justified in using "accepted remedies", unless his patient specifically consents to the use of an "experimental" remedy.[60] This statement has seemed reactionary and unreasonable to doctors, but if one puts it in the context of general doctrine

---

[59] Calabresi, *The Cost of Accidents: An Economic and Legal Analysis* (1970).

[60] Slater v. Baker, 2 Wils. K. B. 359, 95 Eng. Rep. 860 (1767); Carpenter v. Blake, 60 Barb. N.Y. 488 (1871); Langford v. Kosterlitz, 107 Cal. App. 175, 290 P. 80 (1930); *Syr. L. Rev.*, supra note 1, at 1069-1071.

one might say that its teeth are quite effectively drawn. General principles require the consent of the patient to any therapy, usual or unusual. It is just that as the therapy moves away from the standard and the accepted, the need for explicit consent, full disclosure of risks and alternatives, becomes more acute, and more likely to pose an issue. The doctor who prescribes an accepted remedy, under the principles set forth so far, might have a good defense to the claim that he should have told his client about alternative, untried or experimental remedies.[61]

The obligation to advise the patient of alternative therapies does not extend to all the hypothetical, untried or experimental remedies that various researchers are in the process of developing. Where, however, the therapy used is itself experimental, then this fact and the existence of either alternatives or professional doubts become material facts, which like all material facts should be disclosed.[62] Beyond this, where the experimentation is truly and exclusively therapeutic, there are no particular legal constraints that do not apply to the practice of medicine generally.[63] It is simply that the implication of those general doctrines may take on a special coloring in this context.

2.3.3. *Mixed therapeutic and non-therapeutic research: the problem of the randomized clinical trial*

The kind of medical experimentation which causes the greatest legal and ethical perplexities is what might be called mixed therapeutic and non-therapeutic experimentation: The patient is indeed being treated for a particular illness, and a serious effort is being made to cure him. The systems of treatment, however, are not

---

[61] Fortner v. Koch, supra note 49; Curran, "Governmental Regulation of the Use of Human Subjects in Medical Research" in *Daedalus*.

[62] See authorities cited in note 24 supra and accompanying text.

[63] There may come a point, of course, where the procedure is so risky, the benefits so uncertain, and the basis of the treatment so speculative that to use it even with consent is tantamount to unprofessional conduct and quackery. The vagueness of the boundary is, of course, a cause for disquiet for practitioners working with new therapies.

chosen solely with the view to curing the particular patient of his particular ills. Rather, the treatment takes place in the context of an experiment or a research program to test new procedures, or to compare the efficacy of various established procedures.[64] Nor is it the case that this research purpose is limited to carefully reporting the results of treatments in particular cases. Rather, therapies are tried, continued or varied, and patients are assigned to treatment categories partially in response to the needs of the research design, i.e. not exclusively by considering the particular patient's needs at the particular time. Usually it will be the case that there is genuine doubt about which is the best treatment, or the best treatment modality, so that the doctors participating in the experiment do not believe they are compromising the interests of their patients.[65] Or where this is not completely true, it is often the case that no serious nor irreversible harms or risk are imposed in pursuing the research design rather than pursuing single-mindedly the interests of the particular patient. The clearest case, and the one which is the focus of our concern in this essay, is the randomized clinical trial (RCT), in which patients are assigned to treatment categories by some randomizing device, with the thought that in this way any bias of the experimenter and any

---

[64] See authorities collected at Katz, supra note 1, at 376–79; A. L. Cochrane, *Effectiveness and Efficiency* (1972); Chalmers, "Controlled Studies in Clinical Cancer Research," 287 *N. Engl. J. Med.* 75 (July 13, 1972); Shaw and Chalmers, "Ethics in Cooperative Trials" in *Annals*; Veterans Administration Cooperative Study Group, "Effects of Treatment on Morbidity in Hypertension" 213 *J.A.M.A.* 1143 (1970); also reported in Freis et al., *Anti-Hypertensive Therapy — Principles and Practice* (F. Gross, ed. 1966). For discussions of other RCT's such as the comparison of more and less radical surgery in the case of cancer of the breast, see Chapters 3 and 6.

[65] Chalmers, "The Ethics of Randomization as a Decision Making Technique and the Problem of Informed Consent," in *USDHEW Report of the 14th Annual Conference of Cardiovascular Training Grant Program Directors, National Heart Inst.* (1967); Chalmers, supra; Shaw and Chalmers, supra; Cochrane, supra; Chalmers, "When Should Randomization Begin" *The Lancet* 858 (April 20, 1968); Moore, "Ethical Boundaries in Initial Clinical Trials" in *Daedalus*; Mather et al., "Acute Myocardial Infarction, Home and Hospital Treatment" *B. Med. J.* 334 (August 7, 1971); Rutstein, "The Ethical Design of Human Experimentation" in *Daedalus*.

unsuspected interfering factor can be eliminated by the statistical method used.[66] And generally it is said that the alternative therapies between which patients are randomized both have a great deal to recommend them, so that there is no real sense in which one or the other group is being deliberately disadvantaged — at least until the results of the experiments are in.[67]

What is the legal status of experimentation having both therapeutic and non-therapeutic aspects? Since there is a general obligation to obtain consent to a therapy, and since that obligation becomes more exigent as the treatment to be used departs from the ordinary and the accepted, there is at least the legal obligation to obtain consent for the use of the treatment contemplated, with full disclosure of the expected benefits and hazards. This much is straightforward, and not peculiar to the area of mixed therapeutic and non-therapeutic experimentation and RCT's. Moreover, as we have seen, a number of courts have insisted that the disclosure made in obtaining consent include a disclosure of the existence and characteristics of alternative therapies.[68] Certainly if the therapy proposed is experimental in the sense of innovative, this fact along with some description of more traditional alternatives should be part of the disclosure.

The crucial question, and one as to which there is no decided case, asks whether it is also necessary to disclose first that an experiment is being conducted, and second and more delicately the nature of the experiment and the experimental design.

---

[66] See Chalmers and Cochrane, supra; and see generally *The Quantitative Analysis of Social Problems* (Tufte, ed. 1970); Campbell and Erlebacher, "Regression Artifacts in Quasi-Experimental Design" in *The Disadvantaged Child — Compensatory Education*, vol. 3 (1970).

[67] Thus, for instance, in a major RCT of the efficacy of simple as compared to radical mastectomy for cancer of the breast, Sir John Bruce writes: "One of the important ethical necessities before a random clinical is undertaken is a near certainty that none of the treatment options is likely to be so much inferior that harm could accrue to those allocated to it. In the present instance . . . it looked as if the mode of primary treatment make no significant difference, at least in terms of survival." "Operable Cancer of the Breast — A Controlled Clinical Trial," 28 *Cancer* 1443 (1971).

[68] See supra note 25.

Specifically, in the case of the RCT must the doctor disclose the fact that the patient's therapy will be determined by a randomizing procedure rather than by an individualized judgement on the part of the physician? Some physicians active in mixed therapeutic and non-therapeutic experimentation have argued that it is both unnecessary and undesirable to make this last disclosure:[69] It is undesirable because some patients might be scared off, withdraw from the experiment and seek help elsewhere. It is also undesirable because of those patients who, while remaining in the experiment, might be caused such a degree of distress and anxiety that it would interfere with their cure. The disclosure of randomization is argued to be unnecessary since the medical evidence regarding the alternative treatments will often be evenly balanced (that is why the experiment is being conducted — to help resolve the doubts) so that it is in no way inaccurate to tell the patient that medical opinion is divided on the best therapy, and that the patient will receive the best available therapy according to current medical judgements. To tell the patient that he is being randomized, on this view, would add nothing of relevance regarding the expected outcome of his treatment, and thus nothing of relevance to his choice whether or not to consent to the treatment.

There are no authoritative decisions holding that consent in the absence of a disclosure that the patient is being randomized or that his treatment is being determined by reference to factors other than his individual concerns is invalid consent because of incomplete disclosure. The general principle holds that a person must be given all material information relating to the proposed therapy. But is the fact of randomization, or of the existence of an experiment such material information? The information would seem to deal rather with the way in which the therapy is chosen than with the characteristics of the therapy itself. Nevertheless, it would seem that most patients would consider the information

---

[69] See Chalmers, "The Ethics of Randomization as a Decision Making Technique and the Problem of Informed Consent," supra note 67; Chalmers, discussion in *Annals*, at 513–16; Lasagna, "Drug Evaluation Problems in Academia and Other Contexts" in *Annals*.

regarding the choice mechanism as highly relevant,[70] and would feel that they had been "had" upon discovering that they had received or not received surgery because of a number in a random number table. But does this sentiment create a duty; does it mean, for instance, that consent to the treatment was ineffective and the participating doctors are guilty of a battery?

Though there is no authoritative decision to point to, there are analogies from other areas of law which would suggest that full candid disclosure should include disclosure of randomization. The very fact that the doctor acts in the dual capacity of therapist and researcher, and that his role as researcher to some degree does or may influence his decisions as a therapist, would argue that the fullest disclosure of all the circumstances relating to that dual role, and to the basis on which functions are exercised and decisions made would be required.[71] If the relation were not that of doctor and patient, but of lawyer and client,[72] or of trustee and beneficiary of a trust fund,[73] or of a director or officer of a corporation and the corporation,[74] there would be a strict duty to disclose the existence of any interest which the fiduciary has that may conflict with or influence the exercise of his functions in his fiduciary capacity. The fiduciary owes a duty of strict and unreserved loyalty to his client.[75]

Imagine the case of a lawyer for a public defender organization who has agreed to participate in a foundation sponsored research

---

[70] Cf. Alexander, "Psychiatry-Methods and Processes for Investigation of Drugs," in *Annals*; Park et al., "Effects of Informed Consent in Research Patients and Study Results" 145 *J. Nerv. Ment. Dis.* 349 (1967), quoted in Katz, supra note 1, at 690.

[71] Freund, supra notes 1 and 47.

[72] See American Bar Association, *Canons of Professional Ethics*, Canon 6, at 11 (1963). Canon 6 states clearly that the lawyer's duty, within the law is "solely" to his client, and should not be influenced by other interests or loyalties.

[73] See *Scott on Trusts*, § 2.5, 39–43 (3d. ed. 1967).

[74] See Geddes v. Anaconda Copper Co., 254 U.S. 590 (1920) (director); Bingham v. Ditzler, 309 Ill. App. 581, 33 N.E. 939 (1941) (officer).

[75] See, e.g., Guth v. Loft, 23 D. Ch. 255, 5 A. 2d 503 (1939); In re Westhall's Estate, 125 N.J. Eq. 340, 5 A. 2d 757 (1939); People v. People's Trust Co., 180 App. Div. 494, 167 N.Y.S. 767 (1917).

project on sentencing. As part of the research protocol his decision as to whether to plead certain categories of offenders guilty or to go to trial is determined at random. This is intended to discover how that decision affects the eventual outcome of the case at the time of sentencing and parole. His clients are not told that this is how the lawyer's "advice" as to plea is determined.[76]

The law of conflict of interests and of fiduciary relations clearly provides that the fiduciary may not pursue activities that either do in fact conflict with the exercise of his judgement as a fiduciary, or might conflict with or influence the exercise of his judgement, or might appear to do so, without the explicit consent of his client.[77] And if the consent is obtained other than on the basis of the fullest disclosure of all facts not only which the fiduciary deems relevant but which he knows his client might consider relevant, the disclosure is incomplete, the consent is fraudulently obtained, and the fiduciary is in breach of his fiduciary relationship.[78] There is no reason why the doctor should not be held to be in a fiduciary relationship to his patient, and therefore why the same fiduciary obligations that obtain for a lawyer, a money manager, a corporation executive or director should not obtain for a doctor.[79]

However the issue of informing patients of the fact of random-

---

[76] Professor Paul Freund has suggested that it would be improper for a judge to randomize in sentencing. 273 *N. Engl. J. Med.* 657 (1965). Whatever the objection to this may be, it is quite different from the objections I raise in my hypothetical cases or in medical practice. The convicted criminal is not the client of the judge and the judge does not owe him an undivided duty of loyalty. Indeed it is his job to consider social interests in sentencing the individual, and the randomized experiment may be a way of doing this.

[77] See, e.g., In re Schummer's Will, 206 N.Y.S. 113, 210 App. Div. 296 (1924); affirmed In re Schummer's Estate, 154 N.E. 600, 243 N.Y. 548 (1926); In re Westhall's Estate, 5 A. 2d 757, 125 N.J. Eq. 551 (1939); Bearse v. Styler, 34 N.E. 2d 672, 309 Mass. 288 (1941).

[78] See, e.g., Goodwin v. Agassiz, 186 N.E. 659, 283 Mass. 358 (1933); Daily v. Superior Court, 4 Cal. App. 2d 127, 40 P. 2d 936 (1935); Christensen v. Christensen, 327 Ill. 448, 158 N.E. 706 (1927).

[79] Hammonds v. Aetna Cas. & Sur. Co., 237 F. Supp. 96 (N.D. Ohio 1965), motion denied, 243 F. Supp. 79 (1965); Stafford v. Schultz, 42 Cal. 2d 767, 270 P. 2d 1 (1954); Lockett v. Goodill, 71 Wash. 2d 654, 430 P. 2d 589 (1967).

ization might be resolved, it would seem that there is a continuing duty on the part of the patient's physician to inform himself about the progress of the experiment and to inform his patient about any significant new information coming out of the experiment that might bear on the patient's choice to remain in the study or to seek other types of therapy.[80] This is an important issue in RCT's involving long term courses of treatment. If patients abandon one alternative on the basis of early, inconclusive results, no definitive conclusion can be drawn from the trial.[81] Failure to make continuing disclosures and to offer continuing options to the patient in the light of developing information may not constitute the tort of battery, however, since there may be no physical contact requiring a new consent. The wrong which is done to the patient would be in the nature of negligent practice, and as to that the determinative standard is the standard of practice of a respected segment of the profession. The physician who does not keep his patient continuously informed may argue that to do so would interfere with the experiment, and he might find experts to testify that such continuing disclosure in the course of an experiment is not thought to be good practice.[82] The argument should not be accepted uncritically since the practice which the doctor in the case of an RCT would refer to would not be traditional therapeutic practice, but rather the practice of experimentation itself. Indeed it would seem that the doctrine of the case, holding that a physician had a duty to inform his patient that his broken leg was not healing properly and that there was another method of treatment available in a nearby city which was more likely to result in cure,[83] is equally applicable to the case of a participant in an RCT who has been assigned to a treatment category which, as the experiment pro-

---

[80] See supra notes 45 and 46, and accompanying text.

[81] See the discussion of the University Group diabetes trial, discussed in Chapter 6, section 1, for an example of this problem.

[82] E.g., Chalmers, "Controlled Studies in Clinical Cancer Research," 287 *N. Engl. J. Med.* 75 (July 13, 1972); Shaw and Chalmers, "Ethics in Cooperative Trials," in *Annals*; cf. V. A. Cooperative Study Group, supra note 64.

[83] Tvedt v. Haugen, supra note 46.

gresses and the data comes in, appears to be the less successful treatment. Nor would the device, by which only a supervising committee and not the patient's physician has access to the results of the experiment for a determined period of time,[84] insulate the physician from the consequences of this doctrine.[85]

2.4. *Participation in experimentation as a condition of medical treatment*

In Chapter 6 I consider the device of having certain doctors, clinics or hospitals announce beforehand that they would offer treatment only to persons willing to participate in certain categories of research, including RCT's. Would there be any legal objection to such a scheme? Once again in determining this legal question one must rely on conjecture and extrapolation, since there are no determinative decisions dealing directly with this point.

The law is quite clear that an individual physician is free to accept or decline a patient for treatment as he wishes.[86] The only constraint — and it is a serious one — is that once a physician has undertaken treatment of a particular patient, he must continue to treat him according to the best professional standards and may terminate the treatment only if the patient refuses to cooperate in a reasonable manner with him, and even then he has some obligation to see the patient has some other competent alternative to proceed to.[87] Even where the patient refuses to

---

[84] Chalmers, "Controlled Studies in Clinical Cancer Research" supra note 64.

[85] The position I propose here is supported by Zeisel, "Reducing the Hazards of Human Experimentation through Modifications in Research Design," in *Annals*. See also Rutstein, "The Ethical Design of Human Experimentation" in *Daedalus*.

[86] Hurley v. Eddingfield, 156 Ind. 416, 59 N.E. 1058, 53 LRA 135 (1901); *Prosser*, supra note 1, at 341; McCord, "The Care Required of Medical Practitioners" 12 *Vand. L. Rev.* 549, 553 (1959).

[87] Fortner v. Koch, supra note 49; McGulpin v. Bessner, 241 Iowa 119, 43 N.W. 2d 121 (1950); Saunders v. Lischkoff, 137 Fla. 826, 188 So. 815 (1939); *Prosser*, supra note 1, at § 56; McCord, supra, at § 555.

make reasonable payments for treatment, the law is unclear as to how absolute is his right to terminate his care, at least without seeing the patient safely passed on to some public institution that will carry on with the case.

In general in non-emergency situations, there is no duty on the part of a private hospital to admit or treat, so that it may limit care as it sees fit.[88] Those recent cases that have imposed a duty to treat on private institutions in emergency situations, have done so by analogy to cases of negligent termination of gratuitous services. Where a hospital maintains an emergency room, for example, this has been taken as an undertaking inviting the public to rely upon it, and deterring people from seeking aid elsewhere. And in an emergency such a hospital may be obliged to give treatment even if it knows that the patient cannot pay.[89] In one case, an 11-year-old boy entered the hospital for an appendectomy, was given medication, undressed and put into a hospital gown. The hospital later forced the child to leave, in spite of the fact that it was an emergency, when his mother could not immediately pay $ 200. The court found that the hospital had admitted the child (even though official forms had not yet been filled out) and had negligently terminated its services.[90]

By contrast a public institution cannot arbitrarily refuse emergency treatment,[91] so that it would seem to follow that it may not arbitrarily refuse non-emergency treatment either. And there may be a general duty even on the part of private hospitals receiving Hill-Burton funds to provide services (emergency or otherwise)

---

[88] Costa v. Regents of Univ. of Calif., 116 Cal. App. 2d 445, 254 P. 2d 85 (1953) (teaching hospital could limit care); McDonald v. Mass. Gen. Hosp., 120 Mass. 432 (1836); Anno., "Liability of Hospital for Refusal to Admit or Treat Patient" 35 *A.L.R. 3rd* 841.

[89] Wilmington Gen. Hosp. v. Manlove, 51 Del. 12, 174 A. 2d 135 (1961); Le Jeune Road Hosp. Inc. v. Watson, 171 So. 2d 202 (Fla. App. 1965); *ALI* § 323; Comment, "Must a Private Hospital be a Good Samaritan?" 18 *U. Fla. L. Rev.* 475 (1965).

[90] Le Jeune Road Hospital Inc. v. Watson, supra.

[91] Williams v. Hospital Authority of Hall County, 119 Ga. App. 626, 168 S.E. 2d 336 (1969).

to persons who could not pay for them.[92] The courts are split, however, as to whether the Act gives an implied right to poor people to maintain a private civil action to compel hospitals to provide a reasonable volume of services to those who cannot afford them.[93]

From the foregoing it would seem clear that a physician or a private hospital or clinic (except perhaps where the patient entered in the emergency room) could properly make willingness to participate in research programs and particularly RCT's a condition of undertaking treatment. The reason for this is that they have no duty to initiate treatment in the first place. The difficult questions arise in respect to practitioners and institutions that are under an obligation to offer medical care — either by virtue of a prior relationship entered into unconditionally, or because of some special status, as that of a public hospital. May the doctor who has diagnosed and begun treatment of his patient make the patient's participation, say in an RCT, a condition of further treatment? The answer depends on whether the treatment offered constitutes reasonable and proper medical care. In the case of an RCT where the two alternatives both have the status of accepted remedies the very fact of offering one or another is not breach of duty. Indeed it seems clear that the patient has no right to insist on a course of treatment not offered by his doctor or hospital, so long as the treatment offered is itself recognized as proper. To offer only an experimental remedy would not, however, constitute fulfillment of the hospital's or practitioner's duty. Also no prior announcement or condition could dispense either doctor or hospital from their duties of complete disclosure to the patient, as those have been defined above. The issue, of course, is not about the propriety of offering this or that accepted

---

[92] 42 *U.S.C.* §§ 291 et seq. (1946).

[93] Accord, Cook v. Ochsner Foundation Hospital, 319 F. Supp. 603 (D.C. La. 1970); Organized Migrants in Community Action, Inc. v. James Archer Smith Hospital, 325 F. Supp. 268 (D.C. Fla. 1971); contra, Stanturf v. Sipes, 224 F. Supp. 883 (D.C. Mo. 1963), aff'd 335 F. 2d 224 (8th Cir. 1964), cert. denied, 379 U.S. 977 (1965); Ernesti v. Steiner, 327 F. Supp. 111 (D.C. Colo. 1971).

treatment, but about the device for making the choice — randomization. Here I can only guess and extrapolate. If I am right that the normal assumption of a patient should be that a doctor will do his best for him in his individual case, subject only to resource constraints, then it would seem that insisting that a patient participate in a randomized choice of treatment would not meet the practitioner's or the hospital's obligation to provide accepted treatment — the choice mechanism itself being the departure from what the patient is entitled to expect. But this is simply an extrapolation and guess on my part. To make my guess seem more plausible one might ask whether the patient's refusal to participate in the RCT would justify the termination of treatment.

2.5. Statutes and regulations[94]

At present the only relevant federal statute is the Federal Food, Drug and Cosmetic Act § 505.[95] The sections concerning clinical investigation of drugs were added by the Drug Amendments Act of 1962 (Kefauver-Harris Bill). Since § 505 (d) requires that new drugs be proved effective as well as safe, the Act itself has made clinical trials extremely important.

Section 505 (i) requires those doing research into new drugs to inform research subjects or their representatives that a drug is being used for investigational purposes and to obtain the subject's consent, "except where they deem it not feasible or, in their professional judgement, contrary to the best interests of such human being". The FDA regulations implementing this provision state that the person giving consent must be able to choose freely whether to participate in the trial, must be informed about the nature, purpose and hazards of the experiment, including alternative therapies, and must be told of his possible use as a control in a double-blind trial. The regulations also distinguish sharply

---

[94] See generally Curran, "Governmental Regulation of the Use of Human Subjects in Medical Research: The Approach of Two Federal Agencies" in *Daedalus*.
[95] 21 *U.S.C.* § 355 (1972).

between therapeutic and non-therapeutic investigations.[96] The consent of the subject or his representative is always required in cases of non-therapeutic research, and "in all but exceptional cases" of therapeutic research.[97]

Another exception to consent in therapeutic research is when obtaining it would be (in the words of the statute) "contrary to the best interests of the patient". The FDA defined such a situation as occurring when communication of information to obtain consent would "seriously affect the patient's well-being". Professor Curran suggests that the exception had its origins in a hypothetical discussion when the Senate was debating the merits of § 505 (i) — where the patient is ill with cancer but does not know about his condition and obtaining consent to administer the drug would reveal the truth to him.[98]

Since the function of these regulations is to control the distribution of drugs exempted from the FDA's usual regulations by virtue of their being experimental, a manufacturer may have permission to distribute and test such a drug withheld or withdrawn if he does not obtain from each investigator certification that he will follow these guidelines for informed consent. While this is the only sanction in the regulations, it is conceivable that they might also serve to define the standard of care required of those sponsoring and conducting experiments with new drugs in a tort action by an injured subject. This is because courts have been willing at times to adopt standards in legislation[99] or admin-

---

[96] 32 F.R. 8753, June 20, 1967; 21 C.F.R. 130.37.

[97] One example of an exception that may be made is when the patient is in a coma or otherwise incapable of giving consent, his representative cannot be reached and it is imperative to administer the drug without delay. This exception has been criticized on the ground that no one in such a situation should be admitted to a clinical trial. It assumes that there is no other treatment and that terrible harm would result without the drug. If these assumptions are true, the drug should be administered not as part of a research study (and certainly not in an RCT where the subject might not even receive the drug) but purely clinically, since it would be permissible under the law of malpractice to use an experimental drug in a dire emergency if it were believed to be the patient's only hope. See Curran, supra note 94.

[98] Curran, supra note 94.

[99] See, e.g., Martin v. Herzog, 228 N.Y. 164, 126 N.E. 814 (1920); *Prosser*, supra note 1, at § 36.

istrative regulations[100] to specify the meaning of the general standard of reasonable care in negligence actions.

In October, 1973 the Department of Health, Education and Welfare issued proposed rules, designed to protect the rights of experimental subjects in institution receiving DHEW grants.[101] These rules carry forward the DHEW policy expressed in its earlier *Institutional Guide*. No grant or contract involving human subjects at risk (physical or psychological) will be made unless the grantee is affiliated with or sponsored by an institution which assumes responsibility for the protection of the subjects involved by using a medical review committee. This requirement of prior institutional review only applies when a subject is "at risk" in the supported activity. This crucial phrase is defined in terms of "exposure to the possibility of harm — physical psychological, sociological or other — as a consequence of [procedures that go beyond] . . . established and accepted methods necessary to meet [the subject's] needs".[102] It would seem that the *Institutional Guide* had the RCT and the usual argument in its favor in mind, when it goes on to stipulate that even accepted procedures may place a subject at risk "if it is being employed for purposes other than to meet the needs of the subject . . . Arbitrary, random, or other assignment of subjects to differing treatment or study groups in the interests of a [research project], rather than in the strict interests of the subject, introduces the possibility of exposing him to additional risk. Even comparison of two or more established and accepted methods may potentially involve exposure of at least some of the subjects to additional risks. . . ."[103] Thus it seems very clear that any RCT must be subject to review not because it does, but because it *might* expose some of the subjects to additional risks.

---

[100] See, e.g., Major v. Waverly & Ogden, Inc., 7 N.Y. 2d 332, 165 N.E. 2d 181, 197 N.Y.S. 2d 105 (1960); Morris, "The Role of Administrative Safety Measures in Negligence Actions" 28 *Tex. L. Rev.* 143 (1949).

[101] 38 F.R. 27882 (October 9, 1973).

[102] Ibid. § 46.3 (b).

[103] *DHEW, Institutional Guide to DHEW Policy on Protection of Human Subjects*, pp. 3–4 (DHEW Pub. No. (NIH) 72–102, December 1, 1971).

What is considerably less clear is the consequence of requiring this institutional review even in the case of RCT's involving two accepted treatments. It is stated in general terms that prior review of a project by the institution must include an assessment of the rights and welfare of the individual, the appropriateness of methods of informed consent and the risks and potential medical benefits of the investigation. The rules define informed consent as "including" the following elements: (1) A fair explanation of the procedures to be followed, and their purposes, including identification of any procedures which are experimental; (2) A description of the attendant discomforts and risks reasonably to be expected; (3) A description of any benefits reasonably to be expected; (4) A disclosure of any appropriate alternative procedures that might be advantageous for the subject; (5) An offer to answer any inquiries concerning the procedures; and (6) An instruction that the subject is free to withdraw his consent and to continue participation in the project activity at any time. In addition, no exculpatory language may be included, and the consent should be documented.[104]

While it goes without saying that ordinarily a patient or volunteer subject can withdraw his consent, spelling it out in requirement 6 is of significance in the conduct of RCT's for the reason that the investigator may try to keep subjects in the experiment (even though they would prefer to drop out — perhaps to try the alternative therapy) in order to wait for a statistically significant result.

This strong statement appears, however, to be qualified by a note in the *Institutional Guide*, that states "where an activity involves therapy, diagnosis, or management, and a professional/patient relationship exists it is necessary to recognize that each patient's mental and emotional condition is important . . . and that in discussing the element of risk, a certain amount of discretion must be employed consistent with full disclosure of fact necessary to any informed consent".[105] This qualification does

---

[104] Ibid., § 46.3 (c).

[105] *Institutional Guide*, at p. 8. The phrase is a quotation from Salgo v. Leland Stanford Jr. University Board of Trustees, supra note 24.

not apply in the case where there is no therapy, diagnosis or management and the relation is one of "professional/subject" and not "professional/patient". This note introduces a note of confusion, for the delicate problems arise just because the patient and doctor are engaging in research in the context of a program of therapy, diagnosis, or management. Thus all the important cases fall just between the two stools. And even if we were perched firmly on the therapeutic, "professional/patient" stool, just how much latitude and discretion is there? Perhaps the same kinds of cases were contemplated as in the FDA regulations. Finally, it should be noted that neither the rules nor the *Guide* consider whether the subject must be told that his therapy will be randomized, i.e. told of the choice mechanism by which a therapy is arrived at.

Two themes appear and reappear as we consider the legal context of medical experimentation: the contrast between the law of battery and the law of negligence, and the difficulty of determining whether randomization does violence to the duty a doctor owes his patient. These two themes run together when we consider whether a doctor has an obligation to disclose the fact of randomization and whether he is guilty of battery if he does not. For it is the law of battery that grants the status of rights to the interests in autonomy and physical integrity, and the pressures to qualify those rights for the sake of a larger social good are embodied in the law of negligence. The chapters that follow will develop these same themes but will try to arrive at some conclusions of principle. Can one give a coherent meaning to the notions of autonomy and physical integrity, and even if one can, should these notions play a role in a system of medical care where resources are scarce and demand practically insatiable? A review of the law can do no more than raise these questions — partly because the law is incomplete, and partly because it is open to us to judge the law and to change it. So now we must consider what is right in principle.

The concept of personal care

There was a time when a diagnosis of cancer of the breast was even more terrifying than it is now. At the turn of the century the general medical opinion was that the spread of the cancer throughout the patient's body was inevitable, and that this would lead to death, often a painful and lingering death. In 1894 W. S. Halsted, Professor of Surgery at Johns Hopkins developed a radical procedure for removing not only the tumor but the whole breast, a significant proportion of the chest musculature, and a network of lymph nodes extending to the region under the arm.[1] This operation is now a standard response in the United States to a diagnosis of cancer of the breast. There are certainly many cases in which it is successful, in the sense that there is no recurrence of the malignancy and the patient lives out a normal life expectancy. It is, however, also a very traumatic procedure, both physically and psychologically. Recovery and complete healing are often slow, the ability to move the related arm is sometimes impaired, and the patient often feels "mutilated." More recently surgeons in various parts of the world have begun to doubt that such a radical procedure is necessary,[2] and some even suggest that it might be positively harmful, leading either to a spread of the cancer or some destruction of a part of the body's defense mechanisms to it. In

[1] See R. W. Warren et al., *Surgery*, at p. 733 (1963).

[2] See Cope, "Breast Cancer—Has the Time Come for a Less Mutilating Treatment?", 54 *Radcliffe Q.* 6 (N.Y., 1970), reprinted in *Katz*.

Scotland, for instance, a much less radical procedure, known as a simple mastectomy, has long become standard, at least in some circles and in some kinds of cases.[3] Now both the radical and the simple procedure have their devoted adherents. Adherents of the first would consider it almost criminal to fail to take these forceful, radical steps, thereby subjecting a patient to the risk of an agonizing death. The other doctors are about as convinced of the efficacy of their less radical treatment, and add to their conviction their sense of the desirability of sparing the patient what so many consider a needless mutilation.

Teams of doctors in Great Britain[4] and Denmark,[5] hoping to resolve these doubts and finally to do the best by the patients who would be coming through their services over the years, took this step: Women with cancer of the breast of a certain degree of severity would receive either the simple or the radical operation depending on whether the last digit of a number from a random number table placed in a sealed envelope was odd or even. After following women operated on in these experiments the studies all concluded that the radical mastectomy, the standard treatment in the United States, was not more successful than the simple mastectomy: Neither recurrence nor mortality rates were more favorable after the radical operation. And because the patients had been assigned by the random device, arguments that the assignment reflected a bias, that the kinds of patients were not really comparable, or that the skill of the surgery and subsequent treatment varied were considerably undercut. However, the published reports of these studies do not state whether the women knew that they were part of an experiment, that two alternative treatments were being considered for them; and so, of course, the reports do not state whether the women knew about the device by which the

[3] Bruce, "Operable Cancer of the Breast", 28 *Cancer* 1443 (1971), refers to the practice of surgeons in the Southeastern region of Scotland since 1940.

[4] Bruce, supra; Atkins et al., "Treatment of Early Breast Cancer" *Brit. Med. J.* 423 (May 20, 1972). Brinkley and Haybittle, "Treatment of Stage II Carcinoma of the Female Breast" *The Lancet* 291 (August 6, 1966).

[5] Kaae and Johansen, "Simple Mastectomy plus Postoperative Irradiation by the Method of McWhirter for Mammary Carcinoma" 170 *Annals of Surgery* 895 (1969).

treatment they received was determined. If one day it is agreed to make the simple operation the standard operation, it will be thanks to the information gathered in studies like those described. And the participants in those studies who received the radical treatment, after all, received that treatment which most specialists in the United States would consider not only standard but absolutely required. Thus it would seem a great good has been procured and no harm has been done which anyone should complain of. And yet is there not room for unease?

That disquiet, and the larger questions of personal, social and specifically medical ethics implicated in it, are the subjects of the balance of this essay. The legal resolution of these issues can give concreteness and realism to our speculations; it cannot be dispositive. In the end, we must probe the depths of our philosophy to decide what we think is right. If these speculations take us far afield into questions of general morality, the nature of man and of the social bond, it is because such questions interest me as much as does the resolution of the special problems of medical experimentation. Indeed the problems of the RCT interest me here just because they add richness and detail to these most general concerns.

An examination of the ethical issues implicated in randomized clinical trials leads to a widening cone of problems that finally embraces such general and pervasive questions as the conflict between individual rights and the respect for the integrity of the individual on one hand and the furtherance of the welfare of larger groups on the other, the conflict between the rights and claims of identified, present individuals versus the welfare of unidentified, potential or "merely statistical" persons, the conception of the physician as one holding an overriding duty of fidelity to his patient, and perhaps most generally, the appropriateness, and even the possibility of developing well formulated general rules from which can be derived fair guides to the conduct of individual doctors in a large variety of concrete situations. A related set of issues within this widening cone concerns the conception of human welfare which medicine is meant to further. Certainly it is not the case that the physician is simply a disinterested, "pure" scientist

in the sense that his duties and functions are the pursuit of scientific
truth for its own sake. The physician acts in the interest of his
patients — however narrowly or broadly that client group may be
defined — and more particularly their interest in good health. But
the definition of that interest, the definition of good health is itself
in need of clarification and thus philosophical inquiry. The concept
of good health implies a concept of the good life, and the goodness
of life includes a large number of other factors besides simply its
length.

The deepest social and philosophical problems raised by human
experimentation may be divided into two categories: Those that
relate (1) to the conflict between the interests of the individual
patient and his claim to the unreserved ministration of the physician, as opposed to the claims of more or less well defined and
specified wider groups of persons, and (2) to the better formulation
of the interest in good health. I shall first deal with these two
questions separately, so far as possible, and then bring the analyses
together.

3.1. Do randomized clinical trials really pose a dilemma?

3.1.1. The burdens on the experimental subject

The traditional concept of the physician's relation to his patient
is one of unqualified fidelity to that patient's health.[6] He may
certainly not do anything that would impair the patient's health

---

[6] ". . . I will follow that system of regimen which, according to my ability and
judgment, I consider for the benefit of my patients, and abstain from whatever is
deleterious and mischievous. . . ." Oath of Hippocrates, set out in J. Katz, *Experimentation with Human Beings* 311 (1972). This formula may be considered ambiguous
in relation to our subject, as it refers to patients in the plural and the experimenter
may truly believe that he is working to benefit his patients as a class when he determines the choice between two acceptable treatments by a random mechanism as part
of a trial intended to prove which is better. The ambiguity is less in the *Declaration
of Geneva of the World Medical Association*: "The health of my patient will be my
first consideration"; and the *International Code of Medical Ethics* is even clearer:
"Any act or advice which could weaken physical or mental resistance of a human

and he must do everything in his ability to further it. The conduct of a patient's doctor in an RCT appears to conflict with these traditional norms. In this section I shall consider whether a genuine conflict in fact exists, or whether the apparent conflict is not the result of ill formed and incoherent concepts and general principles.

In the RCT a physician (or group of physicians) determines each individual's precise therapy by considering not only that individual's need, but also by considering the needs of the experimental design, that is the needs of the wider social group that will be benefited by a more definitive evaluation of the therapies concerned. Concretely, the actual therapy the patient receives is determined by a randomizing scheme. Does this not, then, clearly pose the dilemma of the physician's duty to the individual and his interest in serving a wider group that would be benefited by the results of the trial? Is this not a case in which that conflict is resolved at least in part by sacrificing the interests and claims of the individual to those of the wider group? Now some would seek to short-circuit this philosophical inquiry at the outset by denying that any conflict exists and that the individual's interests have in any way been sacrificed.

The argument is frequently made that where the balance of opinion is truly in equipoise, there is no sense to the accusation that the prescribing of one or the other of the equally eligible treatments can constitute a withholding of anything or can constitute doing less than one's best (the alternative being no better). And so no one sacrifices anybody to anything.[7] Surely, this is the strongest defense that can be made in favor of the RCT. Yet, this

---

being may be used only in his interest". Quoted in 271 *N. Engl. J. Med.* 473 (1964), and see generally *Katz*, supra, at pp. 311–321.

Cf. American Bar Association, *Code of Professional Responsibility*, Canon 5 EC5–1: "The professional judgment of a lawyer should be exercised, within the bounds of the law, solely for the benefit of his client and free of compromising influences and loyalties. . . ."

See generally T. Parsons, "Research with Human Subject and the Professional Complex" in *Annals* and the quotation from Kenneth Arrow, note 10 to Chapter 4.

[7] In his report of the Scottish breast cancer RCT, Sir John Bruce writes: "One of the important ethical necessities before a random clinical trial is undertaken is a

defense is unsatisfactory at least insofar as it seeks to show that
there is in fact not even any problem to be resolved, no difficulty of
conscience, of ethics and philosophy.

First, one might admit to a certain skepticism about whether the
facts often, if ever, correspond to those which are needed to dissolve so handily the dilemma. Is it ever likely to be the case that
in a complex medical situation the balance of harms and benefits
discounted by their appropriate probabilities really does appear on
the then available evidence to be in equipoise? Or even approx-
imately enough in equipoise to make the argument go through?
I would concede that as to a particular medical condition, even
quite carefully defined, viewed across a general population there
might be a number of cases where the balance between treatments
was equal; but I would suppose that in many of these situations
this equipoise would not exist in respect to a particular patient.
Consider, for instance, the choice between medical and surgical
intervention for acute unstable angina pectoris.[8] I would suppose
that a group of patients could be so defined that the risks and
benefits of the two available courses of action were quite evenly
balanced. But, when a particular patient is involved, with a particular set of symptoms, a particular diagnostic picture and a parti-

---

near certainty that none of the treatment options is likely to be so much inferior
that harm could accrue to those allocated to it". Supra note 3.

Shaw and Chalmers, "Ethics in Cooperative Clinical Trials", in *Annals*: "Our
thesis is that the use of this sound scientific approach in the search for knowledge
has been, and remains, at a low level because of unfortunate and unfounded pre-
judices concerning the ethical propriety of randomization as a technique of the
decision making process in the practice of medicine. In our view the random allocation of patients in a scientific clinical trial is more ethical than the customary
procedure, that of trying out a new therapy in an unscientific manner by relying on
clinical impression and comparison with past experience. . . .

"If the physician (or his peers) has genuine doubt as to which therapy is better,
he should give each patient an equal chance to receive one or the other therapy . . .
each patient must have a fair chance of receiving either the new and, hopefully, better
therapy or the limited benefits of the old therapy".

[8] Editorial, "Coronary By-pass Surgery" *The Lancet*, p. 137 (January 20, 1973);
Auer et al., "Direct Coronary Artery Surgery for Impending Myocardial Infarction"
44 *Circulation* 102 (1971); Vogel et al., "Emergency Vein By-Pass for the Pre-
Infarction Syndrome" 59 *Chest* 606 (1971).

cular set of values and preferences (this last is an issue on which more must be said later), then one may doubt how often a physician carefully going into all of these particularities would conclude that the risks and benefits are truly equal.

Perhaps, after all, this may happen, and may happen often enough to justify a significant number of RCT's. But before one concludes that the dilemma has really been dissolved in these cases, one must be quite careful to determine whether the condition of equipoise obtains just because it has been previously decided not to inquire too closely into the particular circumstances of the particular patient, proceeding rather on the balance of risks and benefits as they pertain to a larger group. One must be careful of this, because if the equipoise appears as a result of this failure of inquiry, then the sacrifice has indeed taken place, but only at another level, in a different way. One might say that the individual patient has perhaps not been sacrificed in the crude sense that the best available treatment has been withheld from him, but he has been sacrificed in that for the sake of the experimental design his interest in having his particular circumstances investigated has been sacrificed. But this amounts to the same thing.

The RCT raises a further conflict between the interest of the individual and that of the experiment: What should the patient be told? Should he be told that he is receiving that therapy which in the judgment of his physicians is the best available in his case, or should he be told more fully that his therapy is being determined by some randomizing device in furtherance of a medical experiment?[9] In the case where the choice between the two treatments is not in equipoise, the failure to disclose the existence of the RCT adds insult to injury since it plainly withholds information which any patient should find relevant and indeed the basis for consider-

---

[9] See Alexander, "Psychiatry: Methods and Processes for Investigation of Drugs" in *Annals*; Fletcher, "Human Experimentation: Ethics in the Consent Situation" 32 *Law and Contemp. Probs.* 620 (1967); Park et al., "Effects of Informed Consent on Research Patients and Study Results" 145 J. *Nerv. Ment. Dis.* 349 (1967), reprinted in *Katz* at 690; Zeisel, "Reducing the Hazards of Human Experiments through Modifications in Research Design" in *Annals*. For legal considerations relating to informed consent, see Chapter 2.

ing a change of doctors. The nondisclosure is deceptive because it fails to reveal that the patient's interests are, to some extent, being sacrificed for the sake of the experimental design and thus, the wider social good. That sacrifice might be the overt one of exposing the patient to the risk of a treatment which in the present state of knowledge is somewhat less favored, or the less overt one of not inquiring fully into his particular circumstances (including his particular value system) in order to determine whether the balance of probabilities is in equipoise in his particular case. There are two justifications for non-disclosure frequently offered:[10]

---

[10] "There can be no argument against the requirement that the investigating physician must obtain completely informed consent from patients taking part in trials which are done for the sake of research and from which they do not necessarily have more to gain than to lose. But I believe that the situation is somewhat different when randomization is carried out because the physician does not know which therapy is better for the individual patients. There are two potent arguments against informing patients with a life-threatening disease that the decision about whether or not he should have a life-threatening operation will be made by chance rather than by clinical judgment. (1) It is not in the best interest of the patients because it seems likely that 9 out of 10 would refuse these studies, and therefore the operation, if so informed. If they were in their right senses, they would find a doctor who thought he knew which was the better treatment, or they would conclude that if the difference were so slight that such a trial had to be carried out, they would prefer to take their chances on no operation. Assuming that there is a 50 percent chance that the operation will prove to be effective, then half the patients who were scared out of the operation by having been asked for their informed consent, would have been mistreated. Furthermore, it is probable that a very sick patient needs to have complete confidence in the fact that his doctor has the knowledge to make the right decisions with regard to his care. In the course of a traumatic illness the loss of that confidence may do great harm to the patient. It is a rare patient who could be expected to be objective enough about his own serious illness to welcome the fact that his physician has not enough knowledge to avoid decisions based on ignorance.

"The second argument against informing patients that the decision to operate or not will be based on randomization lies in the fact that it is not customary in the ordinary practice of medicine to inform patients of all the details with regard to how decisions are made in their treatment. Few patients would be saved by established surgical procedures if the physician and surgeon had to recount in every detail the complications of the operation. The most vigorous advocates of portacaval shunt surgery would be able to do no more operations if they were required to explain to each patient that of the 50 reports in the literature the only controlled studies showed no effects, and all of the enthusiastic reports were totally uncontrolled. The physician must assume some responsibility for making decisions in the best interest of his patients.

(1) that the distress this would cause the patient would be therapeutically undesirable, and (2) that the disclosure would endanger

"Although in my opinion the physician may withhold information from the patient about the exact details of how decisions are made in a randomized study, he must inform the patient of the pros and cons of each therapeutic maneuver under consideration, and he must assure the patient that he will not carry out any therapy that he knows to be wrong. He must inform the patient that he is taking part in a study of a procedure that has not yet been established as efficacious. In other words, the patient should know that he is taking part in a research project and should be free to refuse to take part. And it should go without saying that all physicians concerned in a randomized study must be convinced that the knowledge necessary to make a decision in that patient is not available." Chalmers, "The Ethics of Randomization as a Decision Making Technique and the Problem of Informed Consent" in *USDHEW Report of the 14th Annual Conference of Cardiovascular Training Grant Program Directors, National Heart Inst.* (1967).

"When one is trying to diminish prejudice for or against a remedy, however, it is probably preferable, at least scientifically, for subjects and observers to be kept in the dark. To begin with, patients told that they may receive a placebo may refuse to participate in the trial. If such refusals are few, they need not inconvenience the experimenter or the experiment. But if they are frequent, not only will the trial be prolonged, but the generalizations possible at the end may be seriously limited, in view of the possibly atypical nature of the sample.

"It may be argued that such problems are unfortunate but unavoidable if one is to respect an individual's freedom to say 'No'. Indeed so. But since society hedges in individual liberties in all sorts of other situations, is it not desirable at least to consider the possibility that individual freedom — provided serious harm is not involved — may have to yield at times to the general welfare?

"Placebo trials pose no serious ethical problems for me in most situations: If the true merit and hazard of a new remedy are not established, it is unethical not to perform a proper controlled trial (which may, to be sure, use a standard drug for comparison, rather than a placebo, if such a standard is available). Too often the placebo-treated patients turn out to be the lucky ones in such a trial, 'deprived' only of an ineffective and toxic chemical.

"I do object, however, to such deceit as the use of homeopathic doses of drug as placebo so that patients may be told that they will receive only varying doses of active drug. It also strikes me as unacceptable to disguise the placebo treatment as 'a standard and time-honored remedy that is safe and has been proven to help many people' (true though the statement is!).

"On the other hand, I submit that telling patients they will or may receive a placebo changes the rules of the game, with unpredictable Heisenbergian impact. It is a bit like bugging a jury room to observe the jury process at work. It may be reprehensible to do so without asking consent of the jurors, but who would pretend that the behavior of the jurors will be unaffected by the knowledge that they are under surveillance?" Lasagna, "Drug Evaluation Problems in Academic and Other Contexts" in *Annals*.

the experiment by introducing a disturbing element or even by causing the patient to withhold his consent. Both justifications are inadequate to show that non-disclosure does not sacrifice some interest of the subject. Both justifications beg this question, since they assume that the choice by randomization is proper, and thus they assume that limiting disclosure in order to facilitate this kind of experimentation is proper.

Finally, the failure to make full disclosure is problematic even in the case where the two treatments are really in equipoise for the particular patient, with his particular life plan and physical characteristics. That there is a real problem even here is suggested by the high probability that many patients would surely want to know or would feel deceived if they had not been told.[11] The later discussion will consider in detail the real interests that the patient has in being told even in a true "six of one, half dozen of the other" case. Among other things, I shall argue that the patient has an interest in knowing and thus participating in processes that touch some of his most vital interests,[12] even if we are sure that there is only one rational choice for him to make. Thus, whatever the compensating benefits to the participant in the RCT or to society as a whole, it seems pretty clear that the experimental subject has something to lose, and it is his doctor who is imposing these burdens on him. This does seem to conflict with the conception of a physician as bearing an obligation of undivided loyalty to his patient. It is out of that conflict that our subject arises.

3.1.2. Is personal care a coherent concept?

Another, quite different line of argument seeks to defuse this conflict by showing that there is no *peculiar* problem about randomized clinical trials. Doctors have always had to weigh the interest of one patient against those of another, have always had

---

[11] See Alexander, supra; Park et al., supra.

[12] See Alexander, supra; Park et al., supra; R. C. Fox, *Experiment Perilous 19-20* (1959), reprinted in *Katz*; Jonas, "Philosophical Reflections on Human Experimentation" in *Daedalus*.

to weigh the interests of a particular patient against the interests of a larger group of patients. It is argued that the paradigm of the physician who bears unreserved loyalty to the interests of his particular patient can never have been anything but a myth. Doctors have always had to decide which cases constituted emergencies, so that the real, but less urgent needs of one patient would be sacrificed to the more urgent needs of another. Insofar as the paradigm ever had much force, it reposed on the foundation of hypocrisy. To the extent that the doctor has been able to approach the "ideal" of giving unstinting loyalty to the needs of his individual patients, this has only been possible because of deliberate choices or the semi-deliberate acquiescence in a system the result of which was to limit drastically the number of persons who stood to the doctor in the privileged relationship of patient.[13] Surely it is the greatest hypocrisy to extol the unstinting concern of a doctor for the needs of his patients, when what has made this possible is the fact that an overwhelmingly larger proportion of persons were never allowed to be viewed as patients at all, or to have any considerations for their claims. If it is now felt that there is a dilemma, on this view, it is only because those who have previously been fortunate enough to be the beneficiaries of the (more or less) unreserved attention of the available doctors now find themselves required more and more to share those attentions with vast masses who previously had little claim to them.

It can further be pointed out that social institutions always engage in this weighing of the interests of individuals versus those of groups, only in a more open and palpable way. Such institutions may be relatively small scale institutions such as individual hospitals, or they may be institutions of the most comprehensive sort, including the general government of a nation. These institutions do now make and always have made decisions sacrificing individual

---

[13] See, e.g., O. W. Anderson, *Health Care: Can There be Equity?* (1972); S. Harris, *The American Medical Economy*, Chapter 6 (1964); A. Lindsey, *Socialized Medicine in England and Wales*, Chapters 1, 2, p. 152 (1962); for authorities on the economics of health and its history, see notes to Chapter 4 § 4.1.1. and notes to Chapter 5 § 5.2

interests in various ways. Hospitals perhaps make these decisions in a way that approaches those of the individual doctor: by simply refusing to admit as patients a portion of those needing help, and in a less palpable way by creating priorities of various sorts, even in respect to the group that the hospital does admit as its patients. The general government, which is the limiting case at the other extreme, has an equal relationship and duty by hypothesis to all citizens. In discharging this duty, all kinds of resource allocation decisions are made in the name of greater efficiency, which have and are known to have the effect of denying benefits which particular persons may urgently need.

Those who claim that the traditional conception of the physician's obligation is incoherent would locate the physician in a continuum of sources of help to which an individual person in need will turn. They point out that at no place in that continuum is the traditional paradigm of the doctor–patient relationship a possible or coherent one, and that its incoherence is merely better disguised at the lowest level of the continuum. On this view, therefore, the attitudes, perspectives, and mechanisms for choice employed by some general policy maker constitute the true and coherent model. This is a model of efficient decision-making in which scarce resources are allocated in such a way as to maximize the total return that may be expected from them.[14] All lower level institutions — from less inclusive governmental institutions all the way down to the individual physician — should be seen simply as the agents of this efficiency paradigm, implementing its allocational decisions either by conscious advertence, or (what is more subtle) by more or less unreflecting performance of a role whose structure and expectations have been socially defined so as to lead to the implementation of the overall optimization policy of the general government.

This view would dissolve the dilemma by firmly seizing one horn of it (the efficiency horn of it — the horn that speaks to the obligation to the interests of the larger group) and denying the

---

[14] See note 4 to Chapter 4 and accompanying text.

existence of the other horn altogether. The strong and persistent belief in the existence of the duty of the individual physician to his individual patient is explained away (to the extent that it is not simply dismissed as incoherent and sentimental) as being at best an approximate formulation of the proper role that the general system assigns to individual physicians as a way of achieving efficiency.[15]

The sacrifice of the individual's interests implicit in RCT's would be seen by this argument as simply a special case of the general necessity of responding to the claims of individual persons in the context of an overall conception of the welfare of the group. The individual may be sacrificed in order to provide medical assistance to those whom efficiency dictates should receive it. In the case of the RCT he is sacrificed in order to obtain knowledge, but that knowledge is in turn translated into a more efficient allocation of medical resources.[16] So the two are equivalent. And this equivalence just shows that the asserted dilemma regarding RCT's is a false dilemma, since the RCT is but a special case of the only kind of decision making which is rational, given the reality of scarce resources.

3.1.3. The terms of the conflict: distributive justice and rights

This last, frontal attack on the conflict that many have perceived between the need for medical experimentation and the ideal of personal care is the attack with which I shall deal in the balance of this essay. It questions the very coherence of the concept of

---

[15] This line of argument would be just an application to the physician-patient relation of the general argument that utilitarians make to explain the preference we are inclined to give to friends, to relatives, to those to whom we stand in special relations of various kinds, and indeed to ourselves. See, e.g., Smart, "An Outline of a System of Utilitarian Ethics," in J. Smart and B. Williams, *Utilitarianism—For and Against*, at 50–53 (1973); and the references to Sidgwick, *Methods of Ethics* that Smart gives.

[16] The need for the RCT as a way of providing the information needed as a basis for the rational allocation of resources in a national health service, is the argument of A. L. Cochrane's recent book, *Effectiveness and Efficiency* (1972).

personal care, at least in so far as the obligation of personal care appears to conflict with the responsibility of the doctor to act as the agent of the larger social good — present and future. This attack, which views the rights of and duties to the individual wholly as functions of the greater good of the whole, will lead me to ask two questions in this chapter.

First: Does the notion of distributive justice impose any constraints on the conduct of medicine, medical experimentation and RCT's in particular? This question will be considered in the next section.

Second: If distributive justice is a constraint on the pursuit of the social good is this constraint sufficient to explain the intuitive value we attach to the ideal of personal care in medicine? Is it the case that the sacrifice of the individual to the social good is morally permissible, if only the burden of that sacrifice is fairly distributed?

In order to establish a further basis for the obligation of personal care, I shall seek to show in section 3 that there are values implicated in the relation of personal care as such (indeed in all personal relations) which are not perceived when the benefits that may be conferred in the context of such a relation are disaggregated and considered separately. In section 4 I go on to compare this conception of personal care to some of the familiar approaches of economic and cost-benefit analysis. It is my argument that these either cannot account for the goods of personal care or at least do not help us to evaluate those goods. In Chapter 4 I develop the further thesis that implicated in personal care are not only benefits of the sort these techniques can rationalize, but also rights, and that rights are for systematic reasons beyond the scope of such techniques. An understanding of these rights emerges from a consideration of the goals and meaning of medical care. How these rights are to be systematized and implemented in concrete situations of scarcity and conflict is the subject of Chapter 5. This may take us pretty far afield from medical experimentation. But some of the clearest implications of this general analysis and some of its most specific applications have to do with experimentation and the RCT. It is to that subject that I finally return in Chapter 6.

3.2. *Distributive justice*

This section considers distributive justice as a constraint upon the optimization policy which might lead to the sacrifice of the interests of persons, identified persons, for the sake of the good that could be done to a far greater number of a remote, more vaguely identified group.[17] Insofar as the RCT involves deliberately assigning some persons to a treatment which, overall, or in the particular circumstances of these persons — if those circumstances were inquired into — is not the most favorable treatment, to that extent those persons are being sacrificed in the name of greater knowledge which will be used to benefit future sufferers from that disease, presumably in large numbers. Intuitively it seems unfair to impose the burdens of experimentation on some who do not share fully in the benefits; a violation of their right not to be treated as a means alone, not to be treated as a resource available to other people.[18] But can analysis sustain the judgment that these participants in the RCT have indeed been treated unfairly? That is the question to which I now turn.

There are certain injustices that are so gross that few would try to defend them. That RCT's should be performed on, say, the poor, the ignorant, the incapacitated, or those who happened to come for treatment to Veterans' Administration hospitals, while others received the benefit of a fully individualized treatment, would be grossly unfair. Whether this unfairness is not moderated or indeed removed altogether by other factors — such as the payment of compensation, the provision of a much higher standard of medical care than the participating group would otherwise enjoy —

---

[17] See Calabresi, "Reflections on Medical Experimentation in Humans", in *Daedalus*; Fried, "The Value of Life", 82 *Harv. L. Rev.* 1415 (1969), and *An Anatomy of Values*, Chapter 12 (1970); Schelling, "The Life You Gave May Be Your Own" in *Problems in Public Expenditure Analysis* (S. B. Chase, ed. 1968).

[18] The formulation derives, of course, from Kant. See, e.g., *Foundations of the Metaphysics of Morals* 46 (L. W. Beck transl. 1959). For a modern version and application, see Nagel, "War and Massacre", 1 *Philosophy and Public Affairs* 123, at 134 (1972).

is another question to be considered later.[19] But is it equally unfair to treat quite generally sufferers from certain forms of coronary artery disease in the context of a nationwide RCT today in order to obtain information which will benefit patients in the future? Should we not analogize the present generation of patient to the unfortunate ghetto dweller whose health needs are to some extent sacrificed in the experimental design to benefit the outside world? Is it not unfair to sacrifice the present generation to the future?[20] And just as we would not admit in the second case the argument that after all the sacrificial group is much smaller than the group to be benefited, insisting still on some fair distribution of risks and benefits, should we accept such an argument when made against the interests of those living in the temporal ghetto of the present? It is not necessary to insist upon intertemporality (which in the nature of the case with experimentation will always be present) in order to make this point. Why should the interests of those receiving medical care in fifteen selected general hospitals be sacrificed for the sake of those receiving medical care in all the other general hospitals of the world? (I am, of course, assuming the argument of the preceding section that the RCT does in fact impose a sacrifice on many enrolled in it.)

This is the problem of fairness as applied to experimentation, but it should be noted that it is quite general. Wherever the optimization of some index or set of indices of welfare is taken as the sole criterion for allocational and distributional decisions such unfairness is always possible.[21] Thus, for instance, it might be that, given scarce housing dollars, more units of housing can be put up if we concentrate on urban areas to the total exclusion of rural needs. More houses will be built, more people housed, but those who have the misfortune to live in Appalachia will receive no

---

[19] See Chapter 6, § 6.4.3. For a discussion of insurance and strict liability see Chapter 2, at notes 58 and 59, and accompanying text.

[20] The injustice of sacrificing present to future generations is discussed in J. Rawls, *A Theory of Justice* § 44 (1971).

[21] This argument is fully elaborated in Rawls, *A Theory of Justice*, at § § 5 and 40 (1971).

benefit. They are not exactly discriminated against; it is just that one can get "more bang for the buck" by disregarding their needs. Any conclusion as to the propriety of RCT's requires a clear notion of what fairness means in the distribution of risks and benefits in this area.

Now there is a sense in which sacrificing present patients to future patients, or patients in eight selected general hospitals to all other patients, is different from sacrificing the poor to the rich, minorities to the majorities and the like. The latter cases victimize those who are the victims of general, institutionalized unfavorable treatment in the overall structure of society. Moreover, we may assume that it is the poverty of the poor and the political and social disadvantage of members of a minority which have led to their being chosen as experimental subjects. Assuming that racial prejudice or widely unequal distribution of income constitutes injustice in the basic structure of society,[22] then the singling out of these vulnerable groups to sacrifice them to the interests of the larger society is simply a further example of the injustice to which they are subjected.

But if we assume that the distribution of income and political power within the society is roughly correct, wherein lies the unfairness in choosing some group for participation in an RCT, choosing them either at random or because of some characteristic that makes them particularly apt for such study? Thus, for instance, Veterans' Administration hospitals have been particularly apt places for the conduct of RCT's, because of the comprehensive nature of the records they keep, the fact that patients moving from one part of the country to another could be kept within the experiment, and because administrative coordination between many hospitals is particularly convenient, thus leading to more valid, general results.[23]

---

[22] This term is defined and explicated in Rawls, supra, e.g., at § 2.

[23] See Shaw and Chalmers, "Ethics in Cooperative Clinical Trials" in *Annals*. This article refers to a number of important studies carried out in Veterans' Administration hospitals on hypertension (see Chapter VI, section 1), on anti-coagulants after myocardial infarction and after strokes, on preventive portacaval shunt surgery,

Is there any unfairness, when, in the context of an otherwise tolerably decent and just social, political and economic system, a certain population of sick people are entered into an RCT? Let us assume, in order to pose the question sharply, that they have no real choice about their participation — either because they are not fully informed about the nature of the trial or because no satisfactory alternative treatment facilities are available to them. (The British and Danish breast cancer studies with which this chapter began may provide examples.) In order to claim a distributional injustice in such a context it would have to be argued that it is unjust that certain persons ever be singled out to suffer disadvantage for the benefit of others. It is unjust, even if they were not singled out as a result of some pre-existing improper disadvantage in their socio-economic situation. The injustice consists in the very fact of singling out and sacrificing one group of persons for the benefit of some others. In rebutting the charge of injustice in such cases the proponents of the RCT argue that so long as the participants in the RCT have not been chosen arbitrarily — that is because of some economic or social disadvantage — then it might be said that they have been chosen to participate in the sacrifice not unfairly but at random, as the result partly of a natural lottery which made them apt subjects for study (i.e. sufferers of the particular disease) and in part as a result of a true lottery. And where some must suffer, what could be fairer than to draw straws?[24] Since the risk of being a participant is shared by all and the choice of those upon whom the risk will fall is truly random, where is the unfairness? But is the choice

and on carcinoma of the prostate. See also Zeisel, in *Annals*, at 483; "Part of the trouble derives from the vicious circle that now exists with respect to the main participants in medical experiments. They are now primarily recruited from the temporary or permanent inmates of our public institutions, our Veterans' Administration hospitals, our mental institutions, and, often, our prisons. . . ."

[24] See generally, R. D. Luce and H. Raiffa, *Games and Decisions* (1967). For some historical and theological perspectives, see N. Rabinovitch, *Probability and Statistical Inference in Ancient and Medieval Jewish Literature* (1973); F. N. David, *Games, Gods and Gambling* (1962); Hasofer, "Random Mechanisms in Talmudic Literature" 54 *Biometrika* 316 (1967); Childress, "Who Shall Live When Not All Can Live" 43 *Soundings* 33 (1972).

of those to be disadvantaged by the RCT truly random, and if it is random is that randomness sufficient to obviate any unfairness? In considering these arguments I think we approach the heart of some of the ethical issues relating to RCT's.

The argument that sacrificing this or that convenient group is fair where membership in the group is an arbitrary, natural occurrence should be suspect because it proves too much; indeed it proves everything and anything. It would justify enslaving those who are weaker, despoiling the defenseless, ignoring the suffering of the unfortunate, because in each case these characteristics are acquired arbitrarily, at random. The effect of the argument would be to justify morally any and all burdens which we can in fact succeed in imposing on each other. But that is the very opposite of morality, for morality is concerned to restrain the impulse to profit from natural disadvantage and to require justification for imposing greater burdens on others than we accept for ourselves. But one makes just this kind of immoral argument in arguing that the misfortune of illness is a random event fairly enough distributed to justify imposing even more burdens on the ill. Indeed the whole practice of medicine may be seen as an expression of this moral tendency to overcome the effects of the "natural lottery"[25] without which disease would be allowed to run its course, weeding out the weak and inept. By seeking to overcome the effects of the natural lottery, we affirm each person's equal dignity, the priority of his moral status as a person over his natural status as a sick person or a weak or handicapped person.

Now it is true that where there is a burden or benefit to be shared — particularly when it is an indivisible one — a lottery or random device seems fair. But whatever the arguments for this might be, they assume a starting point, a benchmark of relative equality or at least of a morally satisfactory initial position. When the participants all start out from a position of equality and the chances are themselves equal, then the lottery may justify a result which *ex post* is unequal. The sacrifice exacted in the RCT is exacted in an

---

[25] This term is explicated by Rawls, supra note 21, at p. 15.

unfair lottery, because one did not deliberately and for one's own purposes choose to run the risk of illness; nor did one choose to run the risk of being subjected to a treatment which is less than the optimum treatment in the individual case. Thus the justification for the RCT in terms of the randomness *within* the experiment would only work, if we were also prepared to hold that children, the mentally retarded, the unusually gifted, or twins of persons requiring tissue donations could be called upon on a random basis against their will to make their sacrifice.[26] And if this conclusion makes one uncomfortable, how much more uncomfortable should one be when the circumstance leading to the person's "eligibility" is itself the misfortune of illness?

Indeed the whole notion, so frequently repeated, that the RCT is peculiarly fair because it assigns persons to treatment categories at random rests on fallacy and confusion. It is fallacy to see some fairness in the fact that sickness may be an arbitrary, random event. And it is confusion to claim that the lottery is after all a fair one because in the RCT the treatment itself is distributed at random and the participants in the test do have equal chances of receiving one or the other treatment. For it is not this or that treatment which is the burden, the sacrifice to be justified, but rather the fact that *all* the participants in the trial are disadvantaged insofar as the care they receive is not chosen exclusively out of a concern for their individual well-being, but with regard to the success of the experimental design.

Now all this goes only to show that one must find some way to apportion fairly the sacrifices of the RCT, or at least to find compensating benefits for the burdens so imposed. But would there be nothing undesirable about the RCT if only one could distribute the burdens of the sacrifice fairly? Without doubt the RCT will allow us to come far closer to optimizing our medical resources, to perfecting our medical knowledge. So long as the benefits and burdens of this strategy are fairly distributed, as for instance if all medical care in a society were administered in the context of

[26] See generally, Fried, supra note 17, Chapter 11; B.A.O. Williams, "The Idea of Equality" in *Philosophy, Politics and Society* (P. Laslett & W. G. Runciman, 1962).

RCT's, would anything else be lost? The traditional paradigm of the doctor–patient relation, the ideal of personal care, suggests that what would be lost is just the benefit of being treated with loyal devotion to one's own interests. But is this a benefit to which one is entitled? Admitting that in an RCT one is "used", does one after all have the right not to be used in this way, providing there is no unfairness in the distribution of benefits and burdens? Does one have a right to personal care, even at the cost of certain advantages to all? It is to this question that I turn in the next section and in Chapter 4.

3.3 The good of personal care[27]

This new question raises a far more fundamental issue in respect to RCT's in particular and an optimizing approach to medicine in general. Certainly we must distribute benefits and burdens fairly, but the claim of a right to personal care can justify a waste of resources at best and at worst an unfair benefit to those who happen to be the recipients of this personal care. For it may well be that by pursuing a policy of personal care in respect to those presently before us we actually lessen our ability to help those unidentified persons who will need help later; we may actually worsen their situation. So we must ask whether, once fairness is assumed, is there anything to be said for the right and value of personal care? Is it not a costly piece of irrationality? The first question to answer is whether there is any coherent sense to the notion of giving some preference, some intrinsic value to one's relation to the concrete person before one, otherwise than simply as a function of one's obligation to the group as a whole of which this person is a member.

The doctor's preference for his patient might be seen as a special case of the often noted (and deplored) phenomenon that the

---

[27] In developing my ideas regarding this concept of personal care I have been greatly aided by P. Ramsey, *The Patient as Person* (1970), where very similar notions are developed.

plight of identified persons in immediate danger calls forth a measure of effort and even heroism which would generally be unavailable to ward off perils of a similar or greater degree from a larger but unidentified (statistical) group where the measures involved are effective just because they prevent the peril from ever arising.[28] Examples of this would be the heroic efforts to save the victims of mining accidents and the relative lack of concern for measures of general safety that would have prevented the accidents from ever occurring. The familiar predilection for curative as opposed to preventive medicine is another example of this phenomenon. And, of course, the reluctance to subject persons to a therapy about which comparatively little is known, which in the present state of knowledge appears slightly less eligible than another therapy, with the result that the true benefits of the alternative therapy are never better known, is the very example of this preference for the concrete and the immediate which gives rise to this essay. In arguing for the obligation of personal care, I shall by implication at least be defending those attitudes, choices and patterns of behaviour that favor the concrete, the immediate, the identified. But can such preferences even be stated as part of a coherent set of moral principles? To begin with, a number of confusions should be put out of the way.

First,[29] nothing about the optimization view entails that in every conceivable circumstance the impersonal, the preventive, the remote is the more efficient way of deploying our resources. Certainly a concern for overall, long term efficiency makes such moves more eligible, but it may sometimes be that the best thing to do just is to wait until the need arises in its most dramatic and palpable form and then to use all presently available means to meet it. Second, the uncertain promises and disasters of the future are not reason to prefer the immediate *a priori*; rather they are among the many factors that enter into our probability calculus as to the most efficient course of action overall. What we may

---

[28] See Calabresi, Fried, Schelling, supra note 17.

[29] This paragraph summarizes arguments which are fully elaborated in my *An Anatomy of Values*, Chapter 12.

not do is discount the future just because it is the future.[30] Third, although I recognize that immediate, palpable need tends to call forth greater effort (at least until it hardens the sensibilities and leads to cynicism), still we must distinguish between realistically making use of this passion and justifying it as moral and rational on calmer reflection. Fourth, I reject utterly what may be called the symbolic value argument that justifies a preference for the immediate and palpable over the statistical as a way of teaching or symbolizing our concern for the individual.[31] What, after all, is the value we are choosing to symbolize? Is it the value of human life? Then the question arises how exactly are we to conceive that value. Whether to do so in terms of unstinting devotion to the concrete case before us is just the issue to be resolved. Nor do I accept the notion that "we" understand the value of human life and happiness in terms of broader efficiency, but the only way in which "they" can be brought to do their part is to preach the primacy of the concrete. Among other things, by making this argument am I not letting the cat out of the bag, at least to those of "them" who get wind of our argument?

If personal care is to be established as a coherent concept, as a good in itself, no reliance can be placed on the preceding four arguments. At best those arguments show that some practices apparently illustrative of personal care might be referred to an optimizing approach after all. To rely on such arguments would make the good of personal care not an intrinsic good but a contingent good derived from an optimizing point of view and having no validity where optimization does not dictate such an answer. To establish the intrinsic value of personal care, I shall have to argue for the proposition that the relationship of assisting a person in need is an action and a relationship which have a special integrity[32] of their own. They form a unit, a unit of value, and thus may one assert a coherent interest in personal care.

---

[30] On this point, see Fried, *supra* at Chapter 10; see also Rawls, *supra* note 21, at § 45, for a review of utilitarian and economic writing on this issue.

[31] The argument is made both by Calabresi and Schelling, *supra* note 17.

[32] The concept of integrity as it refers to the considerations explored here is used,

To begin with it should be noted at once that many important relationships other than that of doctor to patient make a similar claim as against principles that would require the individual to be judged by and subordinated to the interests of the larger group. For instance, the conduct of friends and family members illustrates familiar and indeed expected loyalty to the interests of one or a small and defined group of persons.[33] It is not only in some emergency but regularly and pervasively that parents are expected to give a special care for the interest of their own children, a care which greatly surpasses any possible claim that might be raised in behalf of a wider group of children or of the population at large. Similarly, the care and devotion that friends show each other can hardly be viewed as deriving wholly from the appreciation that it is just one's friends who stand in the greatest need of such attention. Indeed this narrower focus of our energies and concerns is best illustrated by the concern which we show for ourselves. I very much doubt that I — or very many of us — could justify the amount of time and resources lavished on our own concerns in terms of the proposition that this was, after all, the most efficient of all possible directions for such an expenditure. Although we recognize in varying degrees our obligation and inclination to do our best by our society, or nation, or humanity as a whole, this recognition is generally constrained by an assertion of a right to devote a certain amount of ourselves to ourselves,

---

perhaps for the first time in recent academic philosophic discourse, by B.A.O. Williams, "A Critique of Utilitarianism", § 5 in Smart and Williams, *Utilitarianism —For and Against* (1973).

[33] The utilitarians seek to account for this in terms of the utility of persons concentrating their efforts on those with whom they are in closest proximity. See Smart, "An Outline of a System of Utilitarian Ethics" § 7 in Smart and Williams supra. Needless to say, such an account must be forced to cover the full range of actual felt loyalties. But those in the Kantian tradition with their tendency towards universality and impersonality also fail to give satisfactory accounts of these values. For a strong example, see David Richards, *A Theory of Reasons for Action* (1971). This inability of Kantian theory to account for personal loyalties and obligations is criticized by B.A.O. Williams, in a forthcoming article in which he takes to task not only Rawls and Richards but (quite rightly) my own earlier work, *An Anatomy of Values*, Chapter 12 (1970).

to our families, to our friends. These preferences may, to be sure, be short-sighted and selfish. That is the issue to be explored. That they exist can hardly be doubted.

In doing all that I can for a person in need, I also enter into a special and wholly different kind of relationship with that person from the relationship I enter into when I perform services to a large range of persons, some known, others unidentified. It is a relationship which, like that of friend to friend or of a person to himself, cannot be reduced to a special case of some larger general relation in which all men stand to each other. Rather human relationships and the action they entail must be analyzed discontinuously. Doing everything for a person, almost everything for a person, and only so much as some optimizing policy requires, are not simply points on a smooth continuum. Relieving a person in distress is a discrete human gesture like making love; one cannot remove aspects of the action one by one and still be left with the same thing.[34] Since this argument is central to my thinking about values, relations and rights I must say more about it to make it plausible and to contrast it to the familiar modes of analysis which obscure what is crucial here.

The dominant mode of value analysis assumes that a valued action, event or feeling may at least in principle be infinitely disaggregated into smaller and smaller component parts, the value of the whole being just the sum of these atomic parts. The contrary assumption that I make is that there are valued entities which are ultimately complex; ultimately, in the sense that though one may break them down into component parts, and these component parts may perhaps individually be of value, still the value of the constituted whole — those parts arranged according to these principles — is different and greater than the sum of the parts. It would be preposterous, for instance, to suggest that the esthetic value of a piece of music consists of the pleasing quality of the individual tones. Obviously it is their ordering into a related

---

[34] The thesis I argue for here, which is related to some versions of structuralism and gestalt psychology, is the subject of my *An Anatomy of Values*. See especially Chapters 1–4.

whole that is the ultimate unit of value whether or not the individual tones may also happen to have some independent pleasing quality. In an analogous way contacts between persons attain significance and value according to the ordered patterns which they exemplify. The communication of ideas, the expression of friendship (or enmity),[35] a display of humor, the playing of a game all consist of a sequence of gestures performed according to a pattern — instinctual, conventional or contrived — and against a background of beliefs, expectations and feelings. Gesture, pattern and background together make up a complex whole whose separate elements are to the significant human contact as tones, rhythms and harmonics are to the piece of music. Nor is this a rare phenomenon. On the contrary, the great majority of the significant entities in our lives, whether their significance is cognitive, moral or esthetic, are complex entities of this sort.

Returning to the case before us, the issue may be drawn between two views of a valued relationship in which aid is rendered. Those who would disaggregate the relation, would argue that the relation may be analyzed into (1) the material benefits conferred (as if these were themselves susceptible of analysis into atomic elements), and (2) — for those who insist that the personal quality of the relation is important — the benefits of friendship or sociability in the relation. And so these theorists must be committed to the view that if the material benefits were conferred outside of the relationship, say remotely by a stranger or even a machine, while the sociability or friendship were obtained from the known person, why this would be just as good. Indeed, they might go on to argue, this schism would probably be better, for it allows one to choose efficiently those who can best confer material benefits, while taking one's social pleasures where those are most likely to be found. After all, is it so clear that I should want to have say, my doctor or a life guard as a friend; do I really want to enter into a *personal* relation with these persons?

---

[35] The notion that enmity and combat are relations between persons implying forms and limits is developed in Nagel, "War and Massacre", 1 *Philosophy and Public Affairs* 123 (1972).

Now it is precisely my assertion that we do indeed want to enter into personal relations in such cases. I do not assert — it would be absurd — that we want necessarily to enter into relations of friendship or love with them. But this shows that there are other kinds of personal relations than those of friends or lovers or relatives. The position that one might be indifferent between receiving crucial medical aid from a doctor and receiving it from a machine, while turning elsewhere for whatever "pleasures" of sociability are alleged to inhere in the doctor–patient relationship, is a position that, among other things, gravely misconceives the concept of sociability. The significance of personal relations cannot be precipitated out from the many other goods that are pursued in such relationships. It is not as if there were the goods of productive labor, of teaching, of musical performance, of sexual gratification, of competition and challenge on one hand, and the good of sociability on the other. After all, what is this abstract good of sociability? I submit that to split off sociability from the significant encounters in which it occurs is like splitting off speed from running fast or driving fast. Sociability is, it might be said, an adverbial notion; it is a quality that certain interactions have. It is not something that it makes sense to think of split off from those interactions. And the more significant the interaction on other grounds, the greater the potentiality for significance in the personal relations in those interactions. But of course this means that there are many other significant personal relations than those that correspond to the ordinary notions of friendship or love — relations that are less open and pervasive, but as significant in their own right.

In the case of the doctor–patient relation the elements that combine to constitute the significance of that relation include:

—The importance and nature of the interests served by that relation. This suggests that not everything that now falls into that professional ambit necessarily has to. The identification of these interests and of what is distinct about them is discussed in the next chapter.

—The complex of intelligence, knowledge and judgment that is needed to serve these interests. Particularly, as I shall argue, there is the fact that health has different significance for different persons, depending on their life plans and value systems, and the further fact that in some situations the doctor may need to help his patient not so much to realize his life plan as to realize that he must radically revise that plan.

—The expectations and confidence which tradition (maybe only mythology) relates to the role of the physician in our culture. This is not a circular argument: the fact of the expectations is not being used to account for the expectations. Rather my point is that the role of trusted personal adviser and helper is a distinctive and significant one, as a total role and not just for the discrete benefits conferred within it. In different times and cultures the precise outlines and the kinds of functions included within this role may vary. Yet because of the significance of the role it is important that the commitments of that role be honored, even if the role might perhaps have been defined otherwise.[36]

The intuitive notion is one of the integrity[37] of a relationship, and therefore of conduct which meets the conception of that relationship. And so when a doctor does less than he is able for his patient, albeit in the name of the progress of medicine and the welfare of larger numbers of persons, this is disquieting because it does violence to the integrity of a relationship which the patient assumes he is in, and which doctors have traditionally stated they were in. The notion of the integrity of this relationship is, to be sure, a complex one. Even in its most extreme form, I would doubt that it carries with it the expectation that the doctor will do everything conceivable to further the interest of his patient. He will not, perhaps, endanger himself. He will not, perhaps, allow the claims of his patients to overwhelm his whole existence and all other relationships in which he might stand. But these qualifications themselves refer to structures of rights, relations, and

---

[36] For a discussion of the importance of conventional elements in relations, see Fried, supra note 17, Chapter 9.

[37] See supra note 32. The notion of the integrity of relationships is also developed generally by Nagel, supra note 35.

expectations of the same form as his relation to the patient, of the same form as the relation of helper to helped. The best way to conceive of the system of these relationships is in terms of adjacent obligations, adjacent relationships. And the technique for resolving conflicts is not one of weighing up and balancing, but of drawing the boundary lines and the terms of the obligation.

The notion is one of doing unstintingly what it is that one does, though choosing with care the occasions on which one will do it. The notion of doing one's utmost in a system of adjacent relations can be contrasted to a notion in which the doctor conceives of himself as performing only one large scale action, which is acting as the agent of the health care system to the population at large. On this latter view his activity and his target is a population of persons, while in the former case his activity has as its object a sequence of discrete objects who are individual patients. And in that latter case, it is his responsibility not to exhaust his resources before he has attended to the totality of his object, which is the population at large, while in the former case if he has exhausted his resources (or himself) on a particular patient, then those with whom he has not entered into this relationship and to whom he is no longer available have no complaint.[38]

----

[38] *A Penal Code Prepared By The Indian Law Commissioners* (Macaulay) (1838): ". . . Two things we take to be evident; first that some of these omissions ought to be punished in exactly the same manner in which acts are punished; secondly, that all these omissions ought not to be punished. It will hardly be disputed that a gaoler who voluntarily causes the death of a prisoner by omitting to supply that prisoner with food, or a nurse who voluntarily causes the death of an infant entrusted to her care by omitting to take it out of a tub of water into which it has fallen, ought to be treated as guilty of murder. On the other hand, it will hardly be maintained that a man should be punished as a murderer because he omitted to relieve a beggar, even though there might be the clearest proof that the death of the beggar was the effect of this omission, and that the man who omitted to give the alms knew that the death of the beggar was likely to be the effect of the omission. It will hardly be maintained that a surgeon ought to be treated as a murderer for refusing to go from Calcutta to Meerut to perform an operation, although it should be absolutely certain that this surgeon was the only person in India who could perform it, and that if it were not performed the person who required it would die. . . . Mr. Livingston's Code provides, that a person shall be considered as guilty of homicide who omits to save life, which he could save 'without personal danger, or pecuniary loss'. This rule

How these integral actions and relations come about, what their contents are, in what their integrity consists, and the relationships between them are deep problems of psychology and ethics. I will not, because I cannot, offer a general theory for such problems here. At best in the course of this essay I will offer certain partial solutions to specific problems. Nevertheless it is important to give some sense of the notion of integrity in actions and relations, because it is that notion which captures the special dimension of the subject before us. And as a general concept it suggests an important criticism of the standard classical utilitarian view of ethics. On the utilitarian view, what a person does, the relationships he enters into, and the choices he makes are all made with an eye towards a distant global end, which is furthering the greatest good of the greatest number or some such optimizing goal. But, I am arguing here that the ethical life of human beings, the values they perceive and follow, inhere in the concrete actions they perform and the concrete relationships into which they enter. It is these which allow a man to live in the present and to give ultimate, intrinsic value to the things that he does. Traditionally the doctor has seen himself as a person who stands to his patients in a relation that is at least analogous to that of friend or lover. To be sure the relation is less intense and pervasive, but it is analogous because it has its own integrity, and it demands, at least within its more circumscribed ambit, complete and unstinting devotion. More-

appears to us to be open to serious objection. There may be extreme inconvenience without the smallest personal danger, or the smallest risk of pecuniary loss, as in the case we lately put of a surgeon summoned from Calcutta to Meerut, to perform an operation. He may be offered such a fee that he would be a gainer by going. He may have no ground to apprehend that he would run any greater personal risk by journeying to the Upper Provinces than by continuing to reside in Bengal. But he is about to proceed to Europe immediately, or he expects some members of his family by the next ship, and wishes to be at the residency to receive them. He, therefore, refuses to go. Surely, he ought not, for so refusing, to be treated as a murderer. It would be somewhat inconsistent to punish one man for not staying three months in India to save the life of another, and to leave wholly unpunished a man who, enjoying ample wealth, should refuse to disburse an anna to save the life of another. . . ." See also the excerpt from Professor Anscombe to similar effect, set out at length in note 50 to Chapter 5.

over, being a relationship its value is a value for *both* parties to it, doctor and patient, and both parties have rights that arise out of it. Although I have been focusing on the interests of patients in the ideal of personal care, it should be clear that this ideal implies an interest and a right on the part of the doctor as well to maintain the integrity of his activity, to work not as a tool or as the bureaucratic agent of a social system, but as one whose professional activity is a personal expression of his own nature, the relationships he enters into being freely chosen, the obligations freely assumed, not imposed.

The reciprocal of this relation may be better seen if we recall some of the other relationships that make this demand of integrity: friendship, love, family relationships, the relation to one's self are all examples I have mentioned. Nor are all such instances to be found in the realm of relations between persons. The relationship of an artist to his art or a scholar to truth has this quality. It is evident that the artist gives to his art an unstinting devotion which is analogous to the care a doctor gives his patient. And the relation between the artist's art and his other concerns, his concerns as a person, citizen, parent, and so on, are relations of adjacent demands, whose structure must be adjusted in some systematic way, rather than the relation of factors of supply whose price and productivity determine the optimum mix of products from the artist, as if from a business firm. There may not be many other professional relationships which have this quality; some think that the lawyer owes his client that degree of concern, and that the lawyer, like the doctor, is not to be viewed as a businessman selling a product or a bureaucrat allocating a scarce resource.[39]

What the foregoing argument shows is that the concept of personal care is a pervasive one, which grows out of a relation that people can create only in the context of more or less direct contact, and that the actions and ends pursued in the context of such relations are qualitatively different from those pursued outside of them. Finally, we have seen that the distinct character of

[39] See the American Bar Association, *Code of Professional Responsibility*, quoted supra note 6.

those relations, actions and values gives rise to interests not only in those who benefit from them — in this case the patient — but in the benefactor, here doctors, as well. For doctors, like others entering into relations of personal care, achieve in that relation the capacity to perform a distinct kind of service and to pursue a distinct kind of value. And the structure of these relations and values presupposes that they are deliberately entered into, chosen, assumed as obligations are assumed. But there is still a great deal to be made clear before we know how to respond to the claim that personal care may rightly be compromised or attenuated, as in the RCT, to serve the interests of the wider social group. And specifically, we must inquire in further detail what there is about the kind of service rendered by a doctor that makes the relationship in which it is given of such high significance. In the next chapter I turn to both formal and substantive points concerning the special nature of the doctor's relation of personal care to his patient.

Personal care: interests or rights

Suppose that I have made my case for acknowledging a distinct set of intrinsic values inhering in the relation of personal care. Yet none of the conflicting considerations — excessive claims on scarce resources, the need to develop knowledge, the opportunity to procure great benefits for future generations — have been disposed of by my arguments. At most I have shown that violating the expectations or attenuating the nature of the relation of personal care is more costly than might otherwise have been imagined. But the question remains, is this yet not a cost we should be willing to pay? If personal care is no more than an interest which individuals have, then that interest must be balanced, weighed and perhaps overriden by the weightier or more numerous interests of others. If the concept of personal care, however, relates not to interests but to rights, then these conflicts require a different solution. It is to that question that I now turn.

4.1. Economic theory and medical care

4.1.1. Efficiency

Economic theory, and more specifically cost-benefit analysis,[1]

---

[1] See generally W. Baumol, *Economic Theory and Operation Analysis* (2d ed. 1965); Eckstein, "A Survey of Public Expenditure Criteria" in *Public Finances: Needs,*

have in recent years offered the most sophisticated and precise methods for resolving the conflicts of claims and purposes in the field of health policy, as in many other areas. It is, I believe, no exaggeration to state that in recent years rational analysis of policy problems in the health field has been synonymous with the application of economic and cost-benefit methods. In this section I shall argue that these analytical tools, while obviously useful and in many fields possibly dispositive, are inadequate to provide a complete account of what is best, what is right to do for the different persons involved in providing medical care. To be sure, economists invariably preface their analyses with a disclaimer to the effect that they do not purport to dictate goals, but only to show how values that already exist might best be realized, given the conflicts and scarcities that exist; or more modestly still, to show what are the implications of pursuing this or that policy.[2] My quarrel with this disclaimer is not that it is insincere, but rather that it implies that the choice of goals, the identification of values, is a pre-rational process, lacking coherence or analytic rigor. Of course, it is the very purpose of this essay to attempt — with that rigor and coherence which the subject admits of[3] — to explicate the values, the goods and the rights implicated in medical care.

The analytic framework of these technical economic literatures may, without too much distortion, be summarized in the following way: It is the task of the analyst to identify the relevant costs and benefits, and to devise a suitable common measure — which is usually their money value — in which to express them. The task then becomes one of the appropriate aggregation of these costs

---

Sources and Utilization (National Bureau of Economic Research, 1961); Prest and Turvey, "Cost-Benefit Analysis: A Survey", 75 *Economic Journal* 721 (1965).

[2] These distinctions are implicit in much of the literature, and in the literature on medical economics referred to in these pages. For a general statement, see Milton Friedman, "The Methodology of Positive Economics", in *Essays in Positive Economics* (1953). For an application to the health field see Ruderman, infra note 4.

[3] "It is the mark of an educated mind to expect that amount of exactness in each kind which the nature of the particular subject admits." Aristotle, *Nicomachean Ethics*, Book I, iii, 4 (Loeb Library, 1956).

and benefits in order to perform either the descriptive or the normative tasks: to show what the overall value of a particular policy is, or to pick out the "optimal" strategy, that one which maximizes the sum of benefits, less the costs. Performing these tasks is neither trivial nor simple: There are great practical and theoretical difficulties in the identification of the benefits and costs, in the assignment of a common measure of value to them, and in the formulae for aggregating them, particularly when such complications as uncertainty and dynamics of time processes are involved.

The bulk of the standard or, what one might call, the working literature in health economics has concentrated on a relatively small number of values to be maximized.[4] Quite frequently the

---

[4] For an example of this see Ruderman, "General Economic Considerations" in *Qualitative Aspects and Quantitative Techniques*, 96, 115–116 (Reinke, ed. 1972):

"Basic considerations in establishing priorities can be expressed in the vocabulary of mathematics in the simple relationship:

$P = f(M, I, V, C)$, in which

P   stands for relative *priority;*

f   means that the priority is a function of (bears an identifiable but unspecified relation to) each of the other variables;

M   stands for the *magnitude* of the disease or other condition under attack, commonly measured by statistics of mortality and morbidity, alone or in combination;

I   represents the relative *impact* or *importance* of the disease; in the present state of health economics it cannot be measured with precision, and is usually given an arbitrary numerical value based on the relative incidence among children, the aged, and persons of working age, or some similar factors;

V   is the *vulnerability* of the disease to attack by known and available means; like importance, it cannot be measured with precision, so that arbitrary rating scales based on expert consensus must be used;

C   is the *cost* of the proposed activity; it can be measured with a fair degree of accuracy, as can morbidity and mortality.

The specific formulation of these factors is an arbitrary decision but one that should have a common sense basis. In Latin America, the relationship

$$P = MIV/C$$

has been widely used. Naturally a multiplicative formula is likely to produce

benefits to be attained have been identified with the gains in economic productivity associable with reductions of mortality and
morbidity, the costs being the costs in medical and other resources
necessary to affect changes in these indices. There is an analogous
body of literature in the educational field; and indeed some of the
authors are the same. In both cases the approach taken is what has
been termed the "human capital" view of the subject.[5]

Recently more complex and sensitive concepts have been introduced, correcting some of the most obvious defects of the human
capital approach, such as its failure to recognize that length and
quality of life are viewed as benefits[6] quite apart from increased
productivity. Evaluating health policy only in terms of gains to
productivity may identify a range of factors that would be relevant

---

a different ordering or priorities than one based on the notion of additivity
or some other relationship."

See also M. Feldstein, *Economic Analysis for Health Services Efficiency* (1967);
"The Medical Economy", 229 *Scientific American* 151 (September, 1973); H. Klar-
man, *The Economics of Health* (1965); Prest & Turvey, supra note 1; B. Weisbrod,
Economics of Public Health (1961). An interesting analysis of a particular problem,
is Klarman, "Syphilis Control Programs" in *Measuring Benefits of Government
Investments* (R. Dorfman, ed. 1965).

[5] See Mushkin, "Health as an Investment", 70 *J. of Political Economy* 129 (1962).
For the literature in education, see, e.g., Bowen, "Assessing the Economic Contribu-
tion of Education" in *Economics of Education,* vol. 1 (Blaug, ed. 1968); Schultz,
"Capital Formation by Education", 68 *J. of Political Economy* 571 (1960); Weisbrod,
"Education and Investment in Human Capital" 70 *J. of Political Economy* 106 (1962).

[6] "Health services are similar to education too, in that they are partly investment
and partly consumption, and the separation of the two elements is difficult. An individual wants to get well so that life for him may be more satisfying. But also when
he is well he can perform more effectively as a producer." Mushkin, supra, at 131.
It is traditional in the economic literature to classify comfort aspects of treatment,
such as private rooms, as consumption items.

Klarman, in his article on the economic analysis of syphilis control programs,
supra note 4, considers the productivity losses attributable to mortality and morbidity from syphilis, the costs of treatment, and even the cost attributable to the
stigma of having had syphilis in terms of the lower career prospects resulting from
the stigma. In attempting to calculate the value of the discomfort and other "consumer good" type losses, he equates syphilis with psoriasis, and asks how much
people are willing to spend to be helped with the discomforts of that nondisabling
disease. That figure then represents the consumer goods value of the presumed
equivalent disease, syphilis.

to policy makers if human beings were indeed just like a stock of capital goods — i.e. machinery — to be purchased, maintained and replaced as efficiency demands; but the analysis does not take account at all of the fact that the machines themselves, that is people, have preferences in this area as well. Moving from the unarticulated, almost grotesquely statist premises of the first approach, which is concerned with increasing productivity without asking for whose benefit this productivity is being increased, the newer analyses have sought to include a fuller range of goods associated with health within a general individualistic model. By this model the goal is to maximize the preferences (therefore including the individual preferences for length and quality of life) of the members of society, the consumers of health care.[7]

Unfortunately this salutary refinement entails great difficulties of method. How is the value of living out one's life free from the discomfort, say, of asthma or arthritis (even though these in no way reduce life-time productivity) to be measured? And more difficult still, how is this value to be measured against the value that others attribute to their health, or indeed anything else those others prefer? A metric must be found to allow judgments that include both the range of different goods a single individual pursues as well as the systems of goods pursued by different individuals. The traditional analytic move made in economic literature, and only recently being applied to health economics, is to posit that the value of any good whatever (including, of course, the value of avoiding a "bad") is just exactly the price that an individual would be willing to pay for that good. Further, in the standard analysis, society does the best it can (attains efficiency, Pareto-optimality) when individuals are in fact able to purchase, to trade freely in perfectly competitive markets, and thus to obtain precisely that mix of goods at that price which their system of preferences dictates and their resources permit.[8] Where, as is always the case, perfectly

---

[7] For an excellent recent example, see Mishan, "Evaluation of Life and Limb: A Theoretical Approach" 78 *J. Political Economy* 687 (1971).

[8] See F. Bator, "The Simple Analytics of Welfare Maximization", 47 *Amer. Econ. Rev.* 22 (1957) for an excellent, concise introduction to this topic.

competitive markets do not obtain — because of monopoly power, or the inability of markets to take account of some cost, or imperfect information — it is the function of economic analysis to develop and test hypotheses about what consumers would do if such markets existed, and thus to suggest what public policy should seek to accomplish in the absence of competitive markets with a view to approximating the results that would be achieved in such markets.[9] The enormous intricacy and theoretical difficulties of performing such analyses, account for much of the genius and labor that is expended in economic theory.

Now the health field offers a configuration of circumstances that are especially challenging to the economists' ingenuity. Professor Kenneth Arrow a decade ago presented a detailed analysis of why in that field we are very far indeed from having conditions that approximate a free market.[10] Though there may be today a

---

[9] See F. Bator, "The Anatomy of Market Failure", 72 *Q. J. Econ.* 351 (1958). For a discussion of the last factor, the patient's incomplete knowledge, see Arrow, infra.

[10] Professor Kenneth Arrow has identified these special characteristics of the medical care market that make inapplicable the classic theorems of price theory and competitive equilibrium: (1) The demand for medical services is ". . . not steady in origin as, for example for food or clothing but irregular and unpredictable . . . a departure from the normal state of affairs. It is hard, indeed, to think of another commodity of significance in the average budget of which this is true. A portion of legal services . . . might fall in this category but the incidence is much lower (and, of course, there are, in fact, strong institutional similarities between the legal and the medical-care markets). In addition, the demand for medical services is associated, with a considerable probability, with an assault on personal integrity". (2) "The behavior expected of sellers of medical care is different from that of businessmen in general. . . . The customer cannot test the product before consuming it and there is an element of trust in the relation . . . [the physician's] behavior is supposed to be governed by a concern for the customer's welfare. . . . Advertising and overt price competition are mutually eliminated . . . advice . . . is supposed to be completely divorced from self-interest. . . . It is at least claimed that treatment is dictated by the objective needs of the case and not limited by financial considerations". (3) "Uncertainty as to the quality of the product is perhaps more intense here than in any other important commodity. Recovery from disease is as unpredictable as its incidence". "There is little opportunity to learn from our own experience in respect to disease. Moreover, the uncertainty is very different on the two sides of the transaction. Further both parties are aware of this informational inequality . . . . (4) The supply conditions do not approximate those in a competitive market. Entry into

market price for obtaining relief from the discomforts of arthritis or for the resources necessary to allow a particular person to increase his chances of living until the age of 72, under present conditions there is no reason to assume that those prices represent the true social value of such goods. It is entirely possible that if certain subsidies were removed which artificially lower the prices of some aspects of medical care, that people would be unwilling to purchase anywhere near that high a level of care.[11] On the other hand, restrictive practices in the health industry may make the price of some health benefits much higher than they would be in a free market situation, so that the present level of demand is too low an index of what people would be willing to consume in this area.

4.1.2. Distribution

For the variety of reasons that Professor Arrow and others have demonstrated, then, the market price is not an adequate index, even in the economists' terms, of the value of medical benefits. But if there were perfectly competitive markets operating in the field, or if through theoretical ingenuity we could arrive at the resource allocation that would approximate the results of such fully competitive market forces, would we necessarily be satisfied with the result? I submit that one reason we do not have free, competitive markets setting the price and determining the allocation of medical resources is that we are not confident we would be satisfied with the result even if we could cause the market to operate. Consider, for instance, the extensive and growing system

---

the profession is limited by licensing and the high cost of medical education. To the extent the education is subsidized, the subsidies themselves represent a strong intrusion of non-market forces. (5) Pricing practices in the medical profession are universal, characterized among other things by extensive price discrimination by income and a strong insistence on the fee-for-service mode of payment." "Uncertainty and the Welfare Economics of Medical Care" 53 *American Economic Review* 941, 948–54 (1963).

[11] Cf. Zeckhauser, "Coverage for Catastrophic Illness", Discussion Paper, John F. Kennedy School of Government, September 1972.

of government" subsidies in the United States[12] — not to mention
the almost total subsidization of health care in Great Britain.
Surely the premise of such a system of subsidies is that we are
concerned not only with efficiency in the allocation of health care
(particularly the kind of efficiency identified by the technical
definition of economic analysis), but with its distribution.[13] There
is the judgment that if market forces were allowed to operate
freely, then at least the poor, who are forced to spend their resources on every day necessities and who do not have the information and habits of foresight necessary to economize in he
correct amounts to meet their actual health care preferences, would
be left in a socially intolerable situation. Not only would this be
true of the poor, but it might be true of the children or dependents
of those who are not so poor, but do not choose to spend money
on the health needs of their dependents. In short, efficiency considerations must be supplemented by considerations of distribution,
of equity as well.

The standard approach of welfare economics in this regard is
to argue that, in principle at least, distributional goals can best
be met apart from allocation of scarce resources, and that the
attempts to attain distributional goals through in-kind subsidies

---

[12] "Departure from the profit motive is strikingly manifested by the overwhelm-
ing predominance of non-profit over proprietary hospitals". Arrow, supra note 10,
at 950. For a useful recent statistical summary, see USDHEW, *Medical Care Costs
and Prices: Background Book* (1972). In 1970 only 3.7% of all hospital beds were
in for-profit hospitals; in 1971 24.9% of expenditures for physicians' services were
from public resources, as opposed to 6.7% in 1966; and in 1970 6.8% of all payments
for drugs and sundries came from public sources. For a comparative study of government participation in health in the United States, Great Britain and Sweden, see
O. Anderson, *Health Care: Can There Be Equity?* (1972).

[13] "No individual should be deprived of medical care because of inability to pay,
just as no individual should go hungry or lack adequate housing because of low
income. ... No family should suffer substantial hardship because of the expense
of unpredictable illness or accident". Feldstein, "A New Approach to National
Health Insurance" 23 *Public Interest* 93 (Spring, 1971). See also Arrow, supra note
10: "Charity treatment in one form or another does exist because of this tradition
about human rights to adequate medical care" at 950. The idea is related perhaps to
Richard Musgrave's theory of "merit wants". See Musgrave, *The Theory of Public
Finance*, 13–14 (1959).

is always, at least, a second best,[14] since the allocational ineffi-
ciencies resulting from in-kind subsidies mean that there will be
less to distribute overall, and thus that we could do better by
everybody without such subsidies. The argument is that distribution should be taken care of by what are known as lump sum
transfers, a good approximation of which might be the negative
and positive income tax, with market forces then determining the
allocation of goods which people purchase with their income thus
fixed.[15] What this mode of analysis implies is that there are no
acceptable ethical judgments about what people receive.[16] Rather
there is the inevitable ethical judgment about the distribution of income in society on the one hand, and on the other hand the technical
judgment about how to attain efficiency in the mix of goods which
individuals purchase with their justly distributed income. Applying
this to the field of health care, it would be argued that perhaps
we should work harder to insure whatever distributive justice in
incomes our social ethics might dictate, but that as to the actual
provision of medical care, like other goods, that should be determined so far as possible by the free play of market forces.

4.2. *The concept of rights*

The foregoing sketch of the solutions proposed by economic

---

[14] The argument is made for in-kind subsidies that although direct money transfers
may in theory be more efficient, in-kind subsidies may be the only form of *politically*
feasible transfer. See Lampman, "Expanding the American System of Transfers to
Do More for the Poor" [1969] *Wisc. L. Rev.* 541; Harmon, "On Comparing Income
Maintenance Alternatives" 65 *Am. Pol. Sci. Rev.* 83 (1971); Musgrave et al., 23
Nat'l. Tax S. 140 (1970); "Helping People Buy Essentials" in *Setting National Priorities — 1974 Budget*, Chapter 4 (Brookings Institution, 1973). R. Posner, in *An Economic
Analysis of Law* (1973), makes this point in respect to public provision of legal services
to the indigent, and G. Calabresi, in *The Cost of Accidents* (1970), pp. 78–80, considers such specific redistributive policies in a number of specific contexts.

[15] See generally R. Musgrave, *The Theory of Public Finance*, Chapter 1 (1959).

[16] "Prejudice apart, the game of pushpin is of equal value with the arts and
sciences of music and poetry". *The Works of Jeremy Bentham*, II, 253 (J. Bowing, ed.
1843).

analysis for resolving the conflicts noted in the previous chapter is necessary to provide the background of my affirmative position, (1) that economic analysis has no theory of rights,[17] and (2) that what we are concerned with is precisely the question of rights in personal care.

4.2.1. Rights and efficiency

I shall not attempt to present even in outline a theory of rights in general. There does not at present exist in the philosophical literature a satisfactory, well elaborated theory. What one must take as a point of departure is a more or less intuitive conception of rights which is best articulated in contrast to the concept of interests or welfare implicit in the standard economic theory I have sketched in the preceding section. In this standard economic theory, things count as interests, goods or values just insofar as they are desired by any member of the relevant society. The task of normative economics is to find some way of maximizing the realization of these goods. The theory of economic efficiency, of Pareto-optimality, sets the outer limit of the goods that it is technically possible for the society to realize. Ethics comes in at the level of distribution — and this distinction is the major revision of modern welfare economics as it criticizes the classical utilitarians[18] — in deciding what the relative positions of the members

---

[17] There is, to be sure, a burgeoning body of economic literature that purports to provide a theory of rights. The point of departure is Coase, "The Problem of Social Cost", 3 *J. of Law and Economics* 1 (1960); and a number of articles by Harold Demsetz: "Towards a Theory of Property Rights", 57 *Amer. Econ. Rev.* 347 (1967); "Some Aspects of Property Rights", 9 *J. Law & Econ.* 61 (1966); "The Exchange and Enforcement of Property Rights", 7 *J. L. & Econ.* 11 (1964). Professor Calabresi of Yale has applied this analysis to law. For a recent example, see Calabresi and Melamed, "Property Rules, Liability Rules, and Inalienability: One View of the Cathedral," 85 *Harv. L. Rev.* 1089 (1972). For a suggestive, critical review of this literature, see Mishan, "Pareto Optimality and the Law", 19 *Oxford Economic Papers* 285 (1967). It is just my point in this section that these writings, insofar as they derive entitlements from notions of efficiency, do not provide a theory of rights.

[18] See, e.g., F. Bator, "The Simple Analytics of Welfare Maximization", 47 *Am. Econ. Rev.* 22 (1957); J. Graaf, *Theoretical Welfare Economics* (1957); E. J. Mishan,

of a society should be to each other in sharing in this maximal possible social product. Whether or not that position should be one of equality, limited inequality, or pure profit from one's natural advantage, and what the meaning of equality should be are thought to be ethical questions, to which the technical analysis can make no contribution. The important point that emerges from this view is that neither economic analysis nor the combination of economic analysis with ethical criteria of distribution assigns any intrinsic value to the enjoyment or realization of any particular good by any particular individual. Particular goods that an individual enjoys are determined merely as a function of (1) what the ethical decision states should be his overall position relative to the rest of the group, and (2) how that individual then chooses to define his good with the share that is thus allotted to him.

The concept of a right, by contrast, states that there is a force to the individual's claim to the particular thing which is the subject of that right, irrespective of considerations of efficiency and irrespective of what the notions of overall fairness in the distribution of income or welfare demand. The intuitive notion of a right is that of a claim an individual can make on the system, the validity of which is not simply a function of some optimizing goal of that system.[19] A right is something which must be recognized; an interest is something which must be taken into account in arriving at a total solution. The furthest that welfare economics has travelled in recognizing rights is just precisely in respect to the one ethical constraint which it recognizes: just distribution. If our conception of just distribution is one, for instance, of equality, then to that extent an individual has a right to an equal share in society's goods. If he is told that it is more efficient under certain circumstances that he should receive less than an equal share, then to that extent his right to equality of treatment has been denied, and it has been denied in the name of efficiency.

A Survey of Welfare Economics: 1939–1959 (1960); R. Musgrave, *The Theory of Public Finance* (1959).

[19] For a very clear exposition of the concept of rights, see Dworkin, "The Original Position", 40 *U. Chi. L. Rev.* 500, 520–24 (1973).

And if, as Bentham thought, equality is simply the surest rule for achieving efficiency,[20] for maximizing the sum of happiness in a society, then it follows that one does not even have a right to equal treatment, since equal treatment is not a claim of the person which must be recognized as such, but a derivation from the concept of efficiency.

The view of rights that I would oppose to this recognizes not just the one general right to a fair share of satisfaction, whatever that might be, but also recognizes rights to specific goods under specific circumstances. Thus, if I have rights to a fair trial, to vote, to speak my mind and read what I wish, these rights must be recognized even if recognizing them is at war with achieving efficiency, and quite apart from whether their recognition is part of my total share of the society's goods.[21] Certainly I acknowledge the existence of a general right to a fair distribution of income, but I resist the notion that it is just a matter of economic convenience whether some people receive their share in goods and services while others get somewhat less goods and services but can vote and enjoy freedom of speech. On the contrary, in a decent society individuals have a number of specific rights — the right to the vote, to freedom of speech and so on — and a general right to a fair distribution of the society's goods as well.[22]

A right is a claim or an interest, then, which has a special status. I would say that recognizing an individual's rights is recognizing those interests or claims which establish his position in his social group, and which that social group may not compromise in the general pursuit of the common good. To make the analogy to a game, there are those rules of the game that define the position of the players, that define what it means to be a player in that game. These basic constitutive rules are analogous to what I think of as the rights of a person against his social group. Then there are the moves, the strategies, the things that happen within that

---

[20] "Everybody to count for one, nobody for more than one." Mill, *Utilitarianism* Chapter 5 at note 7 (quoting and explicating Bentham).

[21] The point is made by Mishan, supra note 17.

[22] See generally J. Rawls, *A Theory of Justice*, Chapter 4 (1971).

game and according to its rules, and these have to do with what in economic theory are thought of as questions of efficiency and just overall distribution. Obvious examples of such rights establishing my position as a person who is a player in the general societal game and as one to whom just distributions are made, are my right to vote, to participate in the processes of government, to liberty of conscience and expression, to be free of cruel or inhuman impositions. What I wish to assert here is that included in that list of rights are rights that relate to the concept of personal care.

4.2.2. Negative and positive rights

It might be objected that including personal care in the list of rights is on its face implausible, because the other rights that I have mentioned and which many would be ready to agree are rights, are negative rights, rights not to be interfered with in certain ways. But they are not rights the realization of which requires positive expenditure of resources. Now I think this argument is simply wrong. The right to vote is a positive right, and its implementation presumably does involve the expenditure of some resources. But beyond that, the distinction between positive and negative rights will not withstand analysis.

The right to a fair trial implies, in the case of indigency, the right to a lawyer, and even without implying such a right, a fair trial is clearly a costly procedure in terms of time and resources.[23] But more dramatically, my right to freedom of speech and of conscience only have bite if respecting those rights is a real constraint on the pursuit of some other social goals. To say that a right is a right only when its recognition puts a spoke in no one else's wheels at all is just to say that there is no such thing as rights. But I accept the lesson of economic analysis that an opportunity cost is a cost too: I accept the conclusion that if respecting my freedom of speech makes it more difficult to pursue some other social good, then my right to freedom of speech is costly, does

---

[23] See Michelman, "In Pursuit of Constitutional Welfare Rights", 121 *U. Penna. L. Rev.* 962 (1973).

withdraw resources from the social pool, just as surely as some right which requires paying over a sum of money to me. To be sure, once we have seen that there is no difference in principle between positive and negative rights, and that the recognition of both categories may be costly to society in its pursuit of efficiency or other goals, we are brought up sharply in both cases against the question of how absolutely such rights are to be recognized, and how such rights are to be ranked and bounded against each other.

As I have said a number of times, I do not have a general theory to answer these questions. Interests are weighed, added up, balanced, set-off against each other. The mathematical and economic mode of analysis is appropriate to interests. What the general intellectual mode for drawing the boundaries of conflicting rights is I cannot say. What I shall seek to do, rather, is to explain why and in what sense there are rights implicit in the concept of personal care, and to show what the boundaries of these rights are, at least in respect to some aspects of medical care and in respect to medical experimentation specifically.

4.3. Personal integrity, the goals of medicine, and rights in personal care

There is the pragmatic argument that whatever efficiency might ideally require, the politics of income redistribution are such that sufficient acceptance for needed redistribution can best be found in partial, specific, traditional and rather dramatic areas. But there is a deeper argument of principle by which such subsidies are seen to express the recognition of fundamental rights — rights of which health care is an important and for our purposes the crucial example (but which include also education, to some extent housing, public order, a system of justice, and indeed an orderly democratic system of government).[24] This argument leads to the eluci-

---

[24] See Michelman, supra.

dation of the notion of rights in personal care. The recognition of these rights, as I have suggested in the previous section, is logically prior to the operation of the market system. They create the underlying conditions in which economic actors develop and maintain a sufficient sense of autonomy and a sufficient sense of confidence in their own systems of preferences and their reasonable ability to realize them to make the economic system work. This view contrasts those matters which are needed to found an individual's conception of himself as a choosing being and to support his continuing confidence in that conception, with those values which he then proceeds to choose from the secure position of human personality thus established.[25] This point is perhaps formally most apparent in respect to the institutions of democratic government. It is these fundamental institutions which make possible the model of a market of autonomous, freely interacting competitive producers and self-defining consumers. That being the case, the establishment of these necessary background conditions cannot itself be derived from and left to the operation of a competitive market system. The determination of the goods included in this conception of the background conditions of autonomous choice, determination of the principles of exclusion and inclusion and the detailed working out of the implications of such an analysis present an intricate task which has hardly begun. My task in this section is only to show how the relations of personal care in medicine involve such fundamental concerns and thus involve rights.

4.3.1. Personal integrity

In most general terms, the goal of health care as it pertains to such fundamental human values relates to the maintenance of the integrity, of the coherence of the human person, with specific reference to the physical substrate of that integrity. The human person identifies himself with his body; he knows that he *is* his

---

[25] Rawls, *A Theory of Justice*, § 67 (1971).

body, that his knowledge of and relation to the whole of the outside world depends on his body and its capacities, and that his ability to formulate and carry out his life plan depends also on his body and its capacities.[26] The doctor's interventions are placed in a special category just because he intervenes at a special point in the system which is the person. In illness, the patient himself, not just some extraneous interest, is threatened. Compare the doctor to the garage mechanic. So long as the person's body and his health are regarded as an asset to be maintained and to be phased out when fully depreciated, the doctor is indeed only a serviceman charged with maintenance of a capital good. But a person's relationship to his body, to his health, is not his relation to his productive goods. Instead it is the person's relation to himself. Although a person may properly be conceived as allocating his life resource to best realize his plan and projects, underlying that conception is the conception of a person who has projects. The person comes logically and morally before the various ends he pursues. And so the doctor does not just help provide the means to get the person where he is going; he ministers to the person who has those ends.

The doctor stands in a special relation to his patient because he ministers to the basic unit which is the person,[27] rather than to the attributes and creations which that person gathers around him in pursuit of his purposes. For the person is his body, and the body's health is the integrity of the person. Although I can appreciate that one would wish to avoid such philosophical depths (or shoals), there is no other way that one can have an adequate conception of what is the person's good, and in what his integrity consists.

[26] For psychoanalytic literature, see Freud, *The Ego and the Id* (1923); S. Fisher & S. Cleveland, *Body Image and Personality* (1958); For philosophical literature, see, M. Merleau-Ponty, *The Phenomenology of Perception* (C. Smith trans. 1962); Sartre, *Being and Nothingness*, Part 3, Chapter 2 (Barnes trans. 1966); M. Scheler, "Lived Body, Environment and Ego" in *The Philosophy of Body* (Spicker, ed. 1970); P. Strawson, *Individuals* (1959); Williams, "Are Persons Bodies?" in *Problems of the Self* (1973).

[27] This is the general theme of Ramsey, *The Patient as Person* (1970).

The two most general aspects of the concept of personality are the ability truly and accurately to attain understanding of the outside world and the ability to formulate and realize the plan of one's life in relation to the outside world. The materials available to an autonomous person seeking to develop and realize his conception of good are his own natural capacities, the resources of the outside world, and the more or less free cooperation of other persons. It is in structuring and elaborating these resources that a person expresses himself and builds a life. Typically, one might say almost naturally, the supporting interaction of other autonomous persons is the highest and the richest resource available to a person. By conceiving of each other as both the instruments and the ends of their mutual strivings, men are capable of building a society of mutual respect and cooperation. This ideal good of what has been called social union[28] gathers its significance from the fact that in such a social union each person's individual self-respect and sense of integrity are fostered and reinforced by the conditions of mutual cooperation in which the value and integrity of others is simultaneously affirmed.

4.3.2. Sickness and death

While this conception of human good does involve striving, and creation involves the overcoming of obstacles, a person's conception of this good must also be realistic. It must accept and work with not only the potentialities but the limitations of the actual, concrete situation. And this is most important in respect to the factors of sickness and death. As death is seen as inevitable, it becomes not the ultimate evil and threat to the life plan and to personal integrity but rather an unavoidable constraint, an element in the total picture.[29] The life one fashions, the good one realizes

---

[28] See Rawls, supra note 25, at § 79.

[29] I present a fuller, more theoretical discussion of this in Chapter 10, *An Anatomy of Values* (1970). There is, of course, an enormous literature. A useful discussion and collection of classical and modern statements, may be found in *Death in Western Thought* (J. Choron, ed. 1963). Of the more recent, specifically medical and psy-

is bounded in time by the fact of mortality. It is no more worthwhile chafing at this fact than at any of the other natural limitations of man's situation. The fact of death is overcome not by seeming to annihilate that fact but by pursuing goods whose effects will outlive the person who pursues them. And, as has been seen in a number of great lives and in innumerable ordinary lives, by limiting life resources, death can give value and preciousness to the expenditure of those resources. Such a conception of death implies a corresponding conception of the doctor's role. Since he cannot remove the constraint of mortality, his function in this respect must be so far as possible to adjust the individual to the fact of this constraint and to loosen the constraint so that it is compatible with a reasonable and rich life plan. This would suggest that it is only one of the physician's duties to retard a premature death; it is as much his duty to help assure that when death does come it is a lucid event, somehow consistent with the life that preceded it. Death should not be an event which, at its approach, trivializes and belies the efforts of a whole lifetime to live fully in realistic contact with the external world of facts and persons.[30]

4.3.3. The function of medical care

It follows from this conception that the doctor's prime and basic function is not so much the prevention of death (which is not in his power) but the preservation of life capacities for the realization of a reasonable, realistic life plan. As in particular cases conflicts arise and decisions must be made between various capacities and between the risk of death and the impairment of various capa-

---

chiatric literature, mention may be made of E. Kübler-Ross, *On Death and Dying* (1969); A. Weisman, *On Dying and Denying: A Psychiatric Study of Terminality* (1972); *The Dying Patient* (O. Brian et al., eds. 1970). See also Showalter et al., "The Adolescent Patients' Decision to Die" 51 *Pediatrics* 97 (January, 1973); Waitzkin et al., "The Communication of Information about Illness" 8 *Adv. Psychosomatic Medicine* 180 (1972).

[30] See generally E. Erikson, "Identity and the Life Cycle", *Psychological Issues*, vol. 1 (1959); *Ghandi's Truth*, pp. 194–195, (1969).

cities, the doctor must see himself as the servant, not of life in the abstract, but of the life plans of his patients. And these will surely differ greatly among individuals and also differ relative to the stage of realization of the life plan in a particular case. When the doctor prepares himself to render service in general, and when society trains and equips the doctor to render such service, both must do so from some conception of what kinds of life plans persons actually have, what the capacities are that persons have for realizing them, and what the realistic, inevitable constraints must be.

On this view one of the most difficult and painful tasks of the doctor is in coping with the prospect of premature death and of disabling illness.[31] It is these, rather than the fact of death, of course, which represent the true threats to realistically conceived life plans. Where there is a risk there must be a chance of loss or failure, and every life plan is to some extent a venture, to some extent a system of more or less calculated risks. The doctor helps to avert or minimize these failures. But where this is not possible he is implicated in a much more delicate process, which is the admission of and adjustment to defeat. A person who learns that he must die sooner than he might reasonably have expected or whose activities and capacities will be significantly curtailed by illness must reformulate to a greater or lesser extent his life plan, his conception of himself; he must change. It is a crucial function of the doctor to assist in this process by intervening so far as possible in the physical changes involved, by informing his patient about the realities of his new situation, and ultimately, by helping him to accept and adjust to these realities.

Cutting across these two related functions is a function of particular significance to the subject of this study. The ideal of human life to which the physician ministers is an ideal of a life fully, lucidly lived, a life whose major events and constraints are accepted and internalized into the structure that a free and thinking man creates of that life. And thus the experiences of illness,

---

[31] See authorities cited supra in note 29, especially Showalter et al., "The Adolescent Patients' Decision to Die".

cure and impending death must also be made into significant events having intrinsic value. Since the physician is deeply implicated in all of these events, however, and since he therefore encounters his patient at the *cruces* of his life, it is essential that this encounter be a social encounter out of whose human and social reality the most can be made. A dramatic but by now perhaps trite example of this point is the so-called "natural childbirth" movement. The physical event which radically alters the structure of the parents' life plan is there made into a significant event, an event which is lucidly lived, rather than a more or less extraneous occurrence to be gotten through or around somehow.

The intervention of the doctor, when he deals with serious illness, is replete with richer potentialities. For whenever human beings impinge upon each other, they may do so blindly, as it were, withholding some part of their human personality from that encounter and thus making themselves *pro tanto* mere inhuman instrumentalities of the other person's purposes, or the encounter may be a human and social encounter in which the full range of human capacities is implicated and complete human respect is shown. It might be, after all, that a patient will treat his doctor like some kind of medicine, like a more or less inanimate object used to arrive at an end. And a doctor might connive in such an instrumental relationship. But I take it to be the goal of a fully human life that important relationships be lived significantly and as human relationships. And this is why the model of the doctor as the supplier of a limited, instrumental service is a serious distortion. It may well be — there is after all a tradition of political economy which so maintains — that no human relationship should ever assume this wilfully truncated, merely instrumental aspect.[32]

---

[32] It is, of course, the Marxist critique of capitalism that labor relationships have this characteristic. For a recent, lucid account of this theory, see B. Ollman, *Alienation* (1971). A good statement of Marx's own views, in addition to the *loci classici*, occurs in Marx, *Early Writings* 120 (trans. & ed. Bottomore, 1963). The question which this tradition has not satisfactorily answered — perhaps the problem is tragic and insoluble — is why this is not characteristic of any complex, technological industrial society, regardless of its arrangements of ownership of the means of production.

That is another matter which I do not care to argue. Whatever the validity of such an all-encompassing thesis, I would certainly insist on this thesis in a relationship that involves an intervention at such a crucial point in a person's life, where there is a bearing on his corporeal integrity, which is a sign and substance of human integrity *tout court*.

4.3.4. Rights in medical care: lucidity, autonomy, fidelity, humanity

The rights implied by this identification of the fundamental concerns involved in medical care may be put under four heads: lucidity, autonomy, fidelity and humanity. These four rubrics converge in the notion of the integrity of the relation of personal care discussed in the previous chapter.

Lucidity. The patient has a right to know all relevant details about the situation he finds himself in. This follows from the significance of the situation of medical care for his understanding of what he is and what he might become. Thus lucidity is not just an instrumental benefit, contingently useful to the patient, to his doctor or to some third persons in maximizing this or that set of goods. It is a constitutive good and therefore a right, since it is crucial to a fully human process of choosing one's good and to the process of choosing what kind of person one will be. To deny a patient an opportunity for lucidity is to treat him not as a person but as a means to an end. And even if the ends are the patient's own ends, to treat him as a means to them is to undermine his humanity insofar as humanity consists in choosing and being able to judge one's own ends, rather than being a machine which is used to serve ends, even one's own ends.

Further, an offense against lucidity denies the patient the opportunity to make out of the significant situation in which the patient encounters the doctor a human encounter, a human relation — that is one in which the parties to the relation may equally engage their major capacities, their capacities for intelligence, choice and affection. Denial of lucidity is a sufficient condition for a relation of dominance, and that in itself is a violation of right.

Autonomy. A patient has a right not only to be free from fraud in the relation of medical care, but free from force, violence as well. Thus if a patient, though fully informed, is subjected to a treatment against his will, this too violates his rights. Similarly if the doctor is forced to perform services against his will, this violates his autonomy. Admittedly, no more controversial philosophical notion exists than of this liberty. The intuitive notion is of liberty to dispose of one's self, that is of one's person, one's body, mind and capacities according to a plan and a conception fully chosen for one's self. The idea is one of being one's own man, and from that position entering into relations of friendship, love, generosity and service. In the relation of medical care this means that both patient and doctor fully define their relation to each other, neither being imposed on as a resource at the command of the other.

Fidelity. Dealings among persons create expectations, reliance and trust.[33] Where each party acknowledges not only that his conduct causes expectations to arise in his counterpart, but acknowledges also that these expectations are justified, that is he ratifies them, then deliberately to disappoint such expectations is a form of deceit. It is a form of deceit which is so clearly identified that it has its own name, faithlessness. Thus, lying is a form of faithlessness because the use of language not only generates expectations, but acknowledges those expectations as justified.[34] There is perhaps usually a conventional element to fidelity. The expectations one acknowledges are rarely specified in full in the particular encounter. Rather there is a more or less implicit incorporation by reference of a whole conventional system of expectations. This is the case in the relation of medical care, where the patient relies and the doctor allows him to rely on a tradition of loyalty to his interests.

---

[33] For a fuller discussion and references, see Fried, *An Anatomy of Values*, pp. 81–86 (1970).

[34] See Aquinas, *Summa Theologica*, II–II, question 110, "Of the Vices Opposed to Truth," where lying is defined simply as a false statement uttered with the intent that it be believed to be true. For a discussion of the strictures against lying in Kant's moral philosophy, see M. Gregor, *The Laws of Freedom*, pp. 150–159 (1963). For various utilitarian writers' views on this issue, and critiques of those views, see authors cited in note 13 to Chapter 5.

Humanity. This is the vaguest of the four concepts. The notion is that over and above a right to be treated without deceit or violence, a person has a right to have his full human particularity taken into account by those who do enter into relations with him. It may be that a man has no right to any affirmative consideration at all, but once he has been drawn into a significant nexus, his wants, needs and vulnerabilities may not be ignored even if his right to autonomy is fully respected and he is treated with complete candor. This too is an important element in the concept of personal care.

Once again I must repeat that I have not even here offered a code of rights relating to medical care. I have only explicated what it is to recognize rights in this area at all, and I have indicated the general notions under which the rights in medical care might be gathered. Quite explicitly I have avoided saying how these values can be implemented, how these rights can be recognized in a world in which resources are scarce and rights conflict. Nor have I said much about the social values involved in providing for the welfare of large groups, which are the values that concern the medical researcher and the medical planner as well as the government official. What I have intimated is that the rationalization of all of these rights and interests into a system is something which no simple optimizing scheme can accomplish. On the other hand, I acknowledge that I have no equally clear alternative. The task of harmonizing rights in conflict is far from done. What I suspect is that this task is a very concrete one, whose accomplishment is deeply rooted in the facts of the particular situation, a task in which prudence[35] plays a large, perhaps the largest part. Certainly no general, abstract *a priori* method is available. For this reason my consideration of the competing rights, of the scarcities and of the need to perceive an overall system will proceed by a fairly detailed account of medical practice, administration

---

[35] Thomas Aquinas, *Summa Theologica* II–II, questions 47–52; "Prudence . . . applies universal principles to the particular conclusions of practical matters. Consequently it does not belong to prudence to appoint the end to moral virtues, but only to regulate the means". 47 art. 6.

and planning in a developed Western democracy. It will be in the context of this account that I shall attempt in the next chapter to put in perspective the rights and values in play. And my most specific judgments and resolutions I reserve for the particular problems of medical experimentation and the RCT, to which I return in the final chapter.

Realizing rights — medical care in general

The discussion in the preceding two chapters did no more than identify a significant range of values, interests and rights implicated in the ideal of personal care. The fact remains that in a world of scarcity personal care for some may mean less than personal care or no care at all for others. And personal care may exclude medical research which would result in preventing suffering and waste of resources on ineffective remedies. Some way must be found to adjust these competing interests. Indeed, whether or not we attend deliberately to the social effects of what we do in providing personal care, those effects will still be there. So it is no good just ignoring the question. What we must attempt is that most difficult of ethical and political tasks, the accommodation of rights. For if we take seriously the concept of rights, then we must not conceive the process of accommodation as one in which rights are just treated as so many fungible goods which are to be traded-off and added up to get some highest sum at the end. But what is the system, then, according to which rights are to be harmonized?

The search for principles of accommodation is imperative for another reason. Individual doctors might be able to pretend that the issue does not exist by just ignoring the systematic implications of their small scale, one by one choices. But as soon as we move away from the immediate provider of health care services and consider the choices facing those who must deploy at more or less long term the efforts and resources for providing these services, the kinds of considerations I have been developing in the preceding chapters seem much more remote. The administrator of a hospital must make staffing decisions, capital improvement decisions, purchasing decisions, decisions concerning the systems and routines to be followed in his hospital. Government officials, whether bureaucrats or legislators, make some of the same kinds of decisions, though at a far greater remove and affecting a larger number of individuals. They also make decisions as to what priority to give research and what kinds of research, how much money should be made available to training and what kinds of doctors to train and most generally of all what should be the overall rate of capital accumulation, thus determining the total resources available as between present and future generations. A hospital administrator may just possibly be able to consider all of the patients in his hospital as "his" patients, but surely this way of thinking is likely to be more of a metaphor than anything else. It is a metaphor, moreover, which is hardly available once one moves to even higher levels of bureaucratic generality. What is the relevance of the values and rights proposed in the previous chapters to the decisions made at these higher levels?

I start with a theoretical argument that our philosophical situation seems to be one in which a satisfactory, overall, theoretical solution to the problem of the particular and the general, of the relation of ethics to social theory, may not be available to us, and such solutions as we can have will emerge from detailed consideration of concrete cases. Perhaps out of a whole host of them a general theory may appear. That is why in this essay I attempt to answer these questions only in respect to the particular case of medical care. In this chapter I suggest some rather general answers in respect to medical care overall, and then more specific ones in the next chapter in respect to experimentation and the RCT. In both cases answering these questions requires at least a schematic account of the actual situation of medical care and experimentation in a developed, western country such as the United States.

5.1. Preliminary speculation : the antinomy of the personal and the social

The conflict I have noted between the recognition of individual rights and the rational working of the system as a whole, between the role of the physician and that of hospital administrators and government officials is not at all unique to medicine. In any larger social group there is a system of significant impingements within the group that do not entail personal relationships, or even actual or possible knowledge of identity. This obvious and pervasive fact is recognized by political theory, while specifically ethical theory has usually focused on the principles of personal relations and thus tended to ignore it. Moreover, the principles and concepts in each domain do not easily translate into each other, if they can be said to be consistent at all. And even the point of demarcation between the realm of the personal and the realm of the general is uncertain, with both ethics and political philosophy treating this boundary as problematic. Consequently not only do we think in ways that are hard to bring together, but also the realms of application of these two systems of thought often overlap, leading to inconsistent results. Writers as far apart as Aristotle[1] and Max Weber[2] have noted this difference, and have noted as well the difficulty if not the impossibility of completely dovetailing the two theories into one general theory.

5.1.1. Political versus ethical theory

Classical utilitarianism seeks to overcome this duality by deriving from and subordinating to the principles relating to general policy the considerations that apply at the personal level. For Bentham, Mill, and their latter day followers the strict rules and obligations of personal morality represent a necessary overstatement of general

[1] *Politics*, 1276 b 41 to 1277 b 24 (Book III A, Chapter 3 in Barker transl., 1946).

[2] "Politics as a Vocation" in *From Max Weber* (Gerth and Mills, transl. 1946), especially at pp. 126–127: "The genius or demon of politics lives in inner tension with the god of love...."

considerations, necessary because of the temptations and difficulties individuals encounter in applying the principle of optimization in particular circumstances.[3] Political philosophy has, of
course, also had a strong counter-current which has sought to
take as controlling the principles established in personal relationships and somehow expand them so that they might apply to the
general and the impersonal. Examples of this might be Rousseau's
political philosophy,[4] perhaps that of Kant, as well as the theories
of various romantic, anarchist and utopian thinkers.[5] Hegel's
theories in this regard are of particular interest,[6] but even an
attempt at characterizing them here would take us far out of our
way. I mention the pedigree of this problem in part to document
my assertion that it is a real problem, and in part also to set the
stage and define the terms for the solution I shall work for. Inadequate, inconsistent and troubling though this duality of the personal and the social might be, it is plain, after all, that we have a
problem which must be resolved, so that in pressing for a solution
we may learn something not only about the particular problem
before us, but about more general issues as well.

I dismiss at the outset the defeatist and irrational proposal that
in the large social context one should not think in these more
abstract, general, aggregate, impersonal terms. This position is
irrational since given the fact of impingement in larger social
groups, the unwillingness to take the general point of view will
just mean that the results will be produced by default instead of by

---

[3] Mill, *Utilitarianism*, Chapter 5; Sidgwick, *Methods of Ethics*, Chapter 7; Smart,
"Extreme and Restricted Utilitarianism" 6 *Phil. Q.* 344 (1956); cf. Schelling, "Game
Theory and the Study of Ethical Systems" 125 *J. of Conflict Resolution* 34 (1968). See
also note 33 to Chapter 3 and accompanying text.

[4] *The Social Contract*, Chapter 13: "I answer that the union of several towns in a
single city is always bad, and that, if we wish to make such a union, we should not
expect to avoid its natural disadvantages. It is useless to bring up abuses that belong
to great states against one who desires to see only small ones. . . ."

[5] For instance, Proudhon, *On Justice*; Kropotkin, *Mutual Aid: A Factor in Evo-
lution*; not to mention various contemporary pop-romantics, such as Theodore
Roszack, *The Making of a Counter-Culture* (1969), or *Where the Wasteland Ends*
(1972); or Charles Reich, *The Greening of America* (1970).

[6] I am thinking particularly of the *Philosophy of Right* (Knox, transl. 1942).

conscious advertence and decision.[7] It would be odd indeed to ascribe any virtue whatever to such an ethic, when the basis of the overall moral system I espouse here is the rationality and autonomy of persons. There is, however, a wholly rational version of this thesis which would hold that whenever a social group gets so large that the interaction between its members no longer can be subject to "personal" control, the group should undergo mitosis just for that reason. This is a position which Plato seems to take in *The Laws*[8] and Rousseau in *The Social Contract*. Since I am defining a social group as one in which willy-nilly there are significant mutual impingements, one might only ask if such small, isolated groups are even possible today, whether or not desirable. At any rate, we all do in fact find ourselves in large social groups requiring impersonal decisions, partially out of necessity, and partially out of a wholly free choice favoring the benefits and opportunities that such larger groups confer on all their members.

Seeing the larger group, with its necessity for impersonal decision making, as a creation both of necessity and of human choice, I would suggest that some of the values that I have posited for the case of personal relations do have application in this general, impersonal context. If the larger, more impersonal structure is the context in which human life must take place; if indeed it is the chosen context for the pursuit of certain human goods, then the values I have been describing would require that each member of the society take over into his own thinking, into his own system of ends and values this choice and this necessity. More specifically, each individual would see himself bound to a whole network of other individuals, even though it is not possible to be in personal contact with all of those other individuals. This network is one whose causality reaches into the future to affect the prospects of

---

[7] It is, of course, a familiar theme in recent analytic theories of collective action that the sum of perfectly rational individual decisions may lead to an overall result that all would find relatively undesirable. See, e.g., M. Olson, *The Logic of Collective Action* (1965).

[8] Book, V, 737 c–d: "The territory should be large enough for the adequate maintenance of a certain number of men of modest ambitions, and no larger. . . ."

persons not yet conceived, just as each individual has in turn been affected by a causality stretching far into the past. And one must acknowledge that those to whom one is bound through this network are, like oneself, human persons, with an equal autonomy, and an equal call on our respect and consideration. The point then becomes to design that network of impingements in such a way that the fabric of this network itself expresses the moral equality, the autonomy and mutual respect of the persons within it.

5.1.2. The theory of democracy

A major thrust of philosophical argumentation for democracy would see democracy as the necessary expression of mutual respect and mutual recognition of moral equality of persons implicated together in a social system. An aspect of democratic theory which has received considerable attention in recent literature relates to the way that this expression of mutual autonomy and respect can be maintained in a nominally democratic system, in which by virtue of its size and complexity crucial decisions are made by bureaucracies and technocracies.[9] That, I would suggest, is our subject. Cutting across many theoretical and ideological differences in this literature is the constant theme that the claim for bureaucratic-technocratic power in terms of efficiency must be evaluated against the costs in loss of actual and perceived participation by all members of the society. And there is a general willingness to sacrifice some measure of "efficiency" in order to preserve or increase the fact and sense of participation. The idea is that each person affected by a decision should be able to exercise some measure of choice about it, so that it becomes a goal of the society for this very reason (among others, of course) to educate its citizens to exercise judgment and choice in a wide variety of areas. But more than this, the acts of participation in the processes of choice should

---

[9] For an excellent recent discussion of this view, which summarizes and gives references to the vast literature, see Tribe, "Technology Assessment and the Fourth Discontinuity The: Limits of Instrumental Rationality", 46 *So. Calif. L. Rev.* 617 (1973).

themselves be seen not as instrumental to the protection of one's interest and the furtherance of one's values, but as significant occasions having an intrinsic value of their own. This means that the forms and the processes of choice should express the mutuality of respect that the processes themselves are meant to further.[10] The occasion for choice itself should be valuable as an occasion for learning more about one's fellow citizens. The understanding that is necessary for proper participation would then be seen as having an intrinsic value which in turn reinforces the civic friendship[11] out of which the participation itself grows. I would recall my discussion of the need to endow with intrinsic value the occasion on which the doctor intervenes in the life of his patient and would suggest that the intrinsic value of participation might be analogous to this.

Granted that the individual might give some intrinsic value to his involvement in impersonal choice and interaction by participating in the process of decision, the question remains: Have I not simply multiplied the number of persons who are placed in the dilemma of choosing between a personal morality and a general, political morality? More concretely, how does this analysis help us with what has been urged above as an anomaly: that the individual physician must give unstinting aid to his patients, while the general system can and must decide at every turn to forgo aid to one category of person in order to help another, and indeed to limit the overall allocation to health in favor of other goals?

5.1.3. What are we entitled to ask of theory?

These two lines of analysis lead to an antinomy with which we must come to terms. I would begin by smoking out an implicit, perhaps unconscious presupposition in certain familiar attempts at systematization and resolution: If only we were to formulate and act upon the correct system of principles, then in some undefined sense everything would turn out well. Or perhaps the assumption

---

[10] The point is developed in detail in Fried, Chapters 7 and 8.

[11] The term is drawn from Rawls.

might be expressed negatively: It is not possible if we have hit upon
the correct moral scheme, that two or more persons acting on the
principles of that scheme should come into conflict. But on reflection it should appear that this is an utterly unwarranted, a childish
expectation. Indeed the systems making this assumption — notably
any single-mindedly teleological system like utilitarianism, hedo-
nism or some other worldly religions — are distinguished by their
fanatic sacrifice of prudent virtue, of sound moral intuition, to
some purported systematizing, unifying goal.[12] Why is it not sufficient that morality tell each of us what to do in order to be re-
sonable, honest and loyal men, without promising also that if only
we are moral then everything else will fall into place? Consider
an actual case from the subject before us. In order to argue for
the doctor's obligation not to deceive and surreptitiously injure
a person who trusts him, do we really have to be able to show that
the sum of suffering will be increased if we violate that obligation?
Does the existence of the obligation really depend simply on the
example we set in violating it, the terror and insecurity that would
arise if the violation were generally known, and so on?[13] Indeed
not. When we say that an action is good or bad in itself we mean

---

[12] See J. Rawls, *A Theory of Justice* (1971) at p. 554: "Human good is heterogeneous
because the aims of the self are heterogeneous. Although to subordinate all our aims
to one end does not, strictly speaking, violate the principles of rational choice . . ., it
still strikes us as irrational, or more likely as mad. The self is disfigured and put in
the service of one of its ends for the sake of system."

[13] This is the approach of utilitarian writers. See Smart, "Extreme and Restricted
Utilitarianism", 6 *Phil. Q.* 344 (1956). For the contrary view, see Harrod, "Utilitarianism Revised", 45 *Mind* 137 (1936); Mabbott, "Punishment", 48 *Mind* 152
(1939); and, of course, Kant, *The Metaphysical Elements of Justice* (Ladd transl.
1965), at 100: "A human being can never be manipulated merely as a means to
the purposes of someone else and can never be confused with the objects of the Law
of things. His innate personality [that is, his right as a person] protects him against
such treatment. He must first be found to be deserving of punishment before any
consideration is given to the utility of this punishment for himself or for his fellow
citizens. The law concerning punishment is a categorical imperative, and woe to
him who rummages around in the winding paths of a theory of happiness looking
for some advantage . . . in keeping with the Pharisaic motto: 'It is better that one
man should die than that the whole people should perish.' If legal justice perishes,
then it is no longer worth while for men to remain alive on this earth."

that it has that quality regardless of the good or bad use to which others will put it.[14] This is not to say that we should not strive for the best possible result, only that we should not expect too much, and that the intrinsic value of what we do may remain regardless of the result.

How much can we expect, though? How much and what? The very posing of the question in this way suggests that the lesson has not been learned and that the attempt is being made to push through the antinomy by main force. We cannot say in general, *a priori* what we can expect the outcome to be of acting decently and humanely. We cannot give an expected value to moral virtue. Who says we should be able to? What we can do is ask in the particular case what are the duties and rights of adjacent actors, in the hope that by more carefully examining the concrete details of the particular case the conception of those rights and duties may be refined. This process of inquiry, which goes by various names — the case method, casuistry, prudence — does not disregard the overall effects of what particular actors do. It considers these, however, as an emergent vector of the precepts it refines. And there *is* a process of refinement. For once the particular right or duty has been stated, it must be reconsidered, its meaning explored as against the impingements of the situation in which it exists, including the impingements of other rights and duties.

Now all this may seem vague and obscurantist. But it is precisely my point that to speak of this process in general is bound to be unsatisfactory. If anything can be accomplished it will (or will not) be accomplished as particular problems are studied and conflicts of principles in respect to them worked through. And it may not work. To overcome the vagueness at this level, to make my claims seem plausible in general would require an equally general overall theory that would resolve these and analogous antinomies not only in medicine, but in housing, in war, in love and sex, in dealing with criminals, in education and art. Well, I have no such

---

[14] See Anscombe, "Modern Moral Philosophy", 33 *Philosophy* 1 (1958); Kant, "Concerning the Saying: That May be Fine in Theory but not in Practice" in Kant's *Political Writings* (Reiss transl. 1970).

general theory, and I do not feel inclined to apologize for that, particularly as I look at what are offered up as examples of such general theories. Rather, I shall proceed to examine in some detail the circumstances of the antinomy of personal care and social responsibility as it relates to medical care and medical experimentation. If such an examination leads to a recasting of the rights and duties of the agents at various levels so much the better.

If it appears how doctors, patients, researchers, subjects, administrators and bureaucrats might all live together more or less preserving their own and respecting each others' integrity, that is surely enough.

5.2. *Two models of the health care system*

In this section I shall seek to convey a sense of the pressures on and interactions between agents at each level of the health care system: (1) the level of the provider of primary care, (2) the hospital or clinic administrator, and (3) the government official. I shall not offer a comprehensive review of the economics or institutional structure of medicine in the United States or any other country. Accounts are readily available in all degrees of detail.[15] Rather I shall go into only so much detail as is necessary to give some sense of the realities of the conflict between personal care and social responsibility, and thus of the realities of the situation in which the rights to personal care must be implemented. It accords best with this limited purpose to present my sketch in terms of the two contrasting models implicit in the antinomy I have been discussing. To what extent can and does the real world at each of the three levels recognize the rights implicit in the

---

[15] For a useful survey, see Anderson, "Medical Care: Its Social and Organizational Aspects — Health-Services Systems in the United States and Other Countries — Critical Comparisons", 269 *New. Engl. J. of Med.* 839 (1963). An extensive bibliography is available in Weinerman, "Research in Comparative Health Service Systems", 9 *Medical Care* 272 (1971). See also Brotherton and Forwell, "Planning of Health Services and the Health Team" in *The Theory and Practice of Public Health* (Hobson, ed. 1969).

ideal of personal care, or can the system be best rationalized in terms of a commitment to optimize scarce resources so as to reduce mortality, morbidity or some other index of welfare in the general population as a whole? For convenience here I shall refer to the first mode of action and decision as the personal care model, the second as the optimization model.

I realize, of course, that reality will not correspond to either model. Indeed other factors such as doctors' desire to maximize their incomes and influence, may account for more of what happens in the real world than either of the two models I have posited. But that is beside the point (or beside my point). I am not concerned with the conflicts that may exist, say, between the doctors' claims to income and status on one hand and the claims of their clients, whether as individuals or as a group, on the other. I am concerned solely with the conflict between two models of service to others: the personal care and the optimization models. I am not concerned here with the conflict of either model of service with a model based on the pursuit by the profession of economic or social advantage. That this is an important, some would say, the dominant motive few if any would deny. And if in the account that follows I ignore such factors, it is not because I imagine doctors are motivated solely or primarily by ideals of service, or that I imagine that conflicts in ideals of service are the only ones they feel. It is just that I am not in this work concerned with such other conflicts, and so choose to present the system in a way that abstracts from them and focuses on what is my concern.

5.2.1. Primary care

The primary provider of general medical care in western countries is the doctor.[16] According to the model embodying the ideal of

---

[16] Of course this need not necessarily be so. The primary provider may be a person with less training than is required of a general practitioner today. What is needed is that this person know enough and have sufficient authority in his dealings with specialists to whom he refers the patient that he can effectively represent the patient and maintain control of the case vis-à-vis such specialists.

personal care this doctor would have the obligation to care for his patient in every way that serves that patient's interests in health.[17] This might include hospitalization or reference to specialists. In the case of reference to a specialist, the specialist would have the same obligation as the patient's first doctor, and would in fact become his doctor in the same way. The only difference might be that a specialist would have an obligation also to report to and consult with the patient's original doctor. In case of a conflict of judgment this should ordinarily be reported to the patient, and the patient be given the opportunity to choose the doctor whose advice he will follow.

In the case of hospitalization, the same general conception would apply in respect to those specialists whom the patient encountered, while all other significant contacts within the hospital would be with persons who acted as subordinates to one or another of the patient's doctors, and who had responsibilities and authority derived from the patient's doctor. On this view the hospital is simply a place in which the patient receives care from his own physicians, who have an unqualified duty to him, and from employees of the hospital as agents of the medical staff.[18]

According to the other, the optimization model, no doctor has any particular person as "his" patient, and no patient has any particular doctor as "his" doctor. Rather patients and doctors encounter each other entirely as parts of a social system. The system has certain designated goals: let us summarize these as to maintaining the useful functioning of the citizenry to the greatest extent possible, subject to budgetary constraints.[19] Complex and

---

[17] See authorities cited at note 6 to Chapter 3 and accompanying text.

[18] "... A central feature of the Anglo-American institution [of the voluntary hospital] (which can now be considered American only, as the British have abandoned the old structure) has been its use as a place for the private practitioner to bring his private patients for treatment, but where he had no administrative or financial responsibilities. In return for this privilege, the doctor usually donated care for the indigent who constituted a majority of the hospitals." Somers and Somers, *Medicare and the Hospitals: Issues and Prospects* 53 (1967). See also W. J. McNervey, *Hospital and Medical Economics*, vol. 1, Chapter 2 (1962).

[19] See authorities cited in note 4 to Chapter 4.

highly sophisticated optimizing analyses will have determined the optimum response in each category of situation, and persons would appear simply as instances of these categories. There would be no surprises, and no case would be unprovided for. If it were determined at a certain point to cease care for a person in particular circumstances, this would not be because of any exhaustion of that person's or of society's resources. Resources would never be exhausted in this way. If the planning had been done correctly all allocated resources (and only those) would in the long run be spent in each category of case and for each element of the category. Of course, it is a concomitant of this that under this model far less than "everything" that might be done for a patient would be done in most if not all cases. And, one would know at the outset just how much would be done in a particular case. There would be no difficulty as to levels of involvement, since at each level the overall plan would dictate what was to be done according to that plan. How exactly money would be obtained for the health care system under this model is a separate question. Whether the monies came from governmental sources, which obtained them through taxation, or from private means, on either assumption the model might still work.

It is at the primary level that the personal care model may coincide most closely with the facts. Or at least the accepted myth is one which at this level coincides most closely with the personal care model. Yet a little reflection and acquaintance with the facts must lead one to conclude that reality departs significantly from the personal care model even at this level. For the model to apply there would, first of all, have to be enough doctors in each locality so that anybody seeking medical attention could get it, and moreover get that amount of medical attention which the personal care model entails. (I will set aside problems of unexpected "runs" on generally adequate personnel. These, like emergencies and epidemics generate their own moralities, which I will not consider here.) Further, we would have to assume that somehow or another these doctors would receive appropriate compensation for their work. Both assumptions are, of course, contrary to fact.

There are parts of the country where there exists an endemic, severe shortage of medical personnel. As a result, in those regions many people receive almost no medical assistance throughout their lifetimes, and a large proportion receive what would be considered grossly inadequate care.[20] Furthermore, even in areas where there are much larger concentrations of doctors, the level of medical care has historically depended to a great extent on the economic and social status of the patient.[21] Only in the last several years has utilization of physicians' services by low income equalled that of high income persons. The most significant gains have been in access to hospital services by the aged poor. The greatest disparities still existing relate to physicians' visits for children under the age of fifteen, where the ratio of utilization by low to high income children was .65 in 1971.[22] These gains by the poor are, of course, correlated with the increase in government programs subsidizing health care, such as Medicare and Medicaid. The percentage of total gross national product spent on personal health care rose from 5.9 per cent in 1965-66 to 7.4 per cent in 1970-71 (the percentage in 1926-29 was 3.6 per cent). The proportion covered by public financing rose in the period 1966-1969 from 22 to 36 per cent of the total, and the greatest part of that increase has been in the financing of health care for the aged.[23] And even with such increases it is still felt by many that there are intolerable gaps in coverage and formidable financial barriers to adequate care.[24]

---

[20] For the most recent survey in the United States, see The Brooking's Institution, *Setting National Priorities, The 1973 Budget*, pp. 222–23 (1973). For a recent survey of the history and present organization of health care in Great Britain, the United States and Sweden, see O. Anderson, *Health Care: Can There be Equity?* (1972).

[21] See Anderson, supra; S. Harris, *The Economics of American Medicine*, Chapter 6 (1964); A. Lindsey, *Socialized Medicine in England and Wales*, Chapter 1 (1964).

[22] *Brookings Institution*, supra, table 7–5, p. 225.

[23] Cooper and McGee, "Medical Outlays for Three Age Groups," 34 *Social Security Bulletin* 10–14 (May, 1971).

[24] Feldstein, "The Medical Economy", 229 *Scientific American* 151 (September, 1973), points out that medical insurance, having contributed to the great increase in medical costs while providing incomplete and shallow coverage, has in some cases made financial barriers to good care more formidable. See generally, Edward M. Kennedy, *In Critical Condition* (1972).

If one compares the American situation to the British National Health Service, which is explicitly designed to overcome the economic barrier to seeking what is considered in the community the "customary" level of care, one discovers some analogous and some different problems. Regional shortages of medical personnel (primarily in rural areas) exist in Great Britain as they do in the United States.[25] Moreover, the system for compensating doctors as well as the system for recruiting and training has led to shortages of medical personnel.[26] This has meant at least sporadic overloading of the existing facilities at every level, from the level of the general practitioner through the level of hospital services.

The coherence of the personal care model is perhaps best tested by the case of the British NHS, where all should receive the same kind of care, irrespective of means. The British case forces us to consider what, particularly in the context of the personal care model, is the meaning of the notion that an individual physician with a panel of 3,000 patients has "too many" patients to be able to take care of "properly."[27] Does this not show that what is "ideal" medical care or even "adequate" medical care is completely relative? I suppose there is a realistic upper limit to the amount of care which a conscientious doctor should give even in the absence of any constraints whatever. People should and if need be perhaps should be forced to spend their time otherwise than in the care of their physician. Whatever the theoretical problem of setting this upper limit, we may be sure that this is one problem with which real life will not often face us.

The problem we are faced with is a situation in which, even where more than 8 % of national income (as is the case in the

---

[25] See O. Anderson, supra note 20; A. Lindsey, supra note 21.

[26] Maddox, "Muddling Through: Planning for Health Care in England" 9 *Medical Care* 439, at 442–43 (1971).

[27] See Lindsey, supra note 21, Chapter 7. The original 1948 regulations of the NHS placed a ceiling of 4,000 on a doctor's list. Some industrial districts had ratios of as many as 5,000 patients to a doctor while in southern England the average was from 1,100 to 1,500 to one.

United States)[28] is devoted to medical care some system of allocation must obtain. And in Great Britain the percentage of a
much smaller per capita income is between five and six percent.[29]
In Great Britain the rationing system at the level of the individual
physician is a combination of queuing and allocation in terms of
seriousness of need. Typically what appears to happen in the
doctor's consulting room in Great Britain under National Health
is that persons not in acute emergencies must simply show up in
their doctor's waiting room and wait their turn, hoping that their
turn will come during consulting hours.[30] Moreover, doctors
themselves appear to adjust the length of the consultation in
terms of the length of the queue. Statistics indicate that as patients'
expectations and behaviour began to take full account of the
free availability of medical care under the NHS, and thus as the
queues increased and the number of patients in each doctor's
panel increased, the average length of a consultation decreased
correspondingly.[31]

I know of no evidence that in American practice doctors have
found any lengthening of the queues for their services. The proportion of physicians to the total population has increased modestly
from 149 per 100,000 in 1950 to 161 per 100,000 in 1968 (the
proportion in Great Britain is far smaller).[32] Perhaps also in
the United States consultations have been shortened and treatment streamlined. Another trend in American medical economics
is the imposition of various costs controls on the amounts to be
reimbursed for various medical services including physicians'
visits.[33] This too would exert a pressure on physicians to increase

---

[28] O. Anderson, supra note 20, Table A6, p. 217. The somewhat different percentage referred to at note 23 is based on gross national product.

[29] Ibid.

[30] Lindsey, supra note 21, Chapter 9.

[31] Ibid. at 214. Lindsey refers to Titmuss' contrary view that "many of the doctors
on an average had more time for each patient, if they chose to use it. . .".

[32] Anderson, supra note 20, at table A15, p. 231, gives a proportion of 119 per
100,000 in 1967, up from 99 in 1950.

[33] See note 36 infra; Egdal, "Foundations for Medical care" 288 *New Engl. J. Med.*
491 (1973); Saward, "The Organization of Medical Care" 229 *Scientific American*
169 (September, 1973); Somers and Somers, supra note 18, pp. 68–71.

their "output" in order to maintain their income, and indeed physicians have more than maintained their incomes.[34]

Does this suggest that the personal care model may be incompatible with an obligation to supply equal or at least adequate medical care to all? Perhaps the personal care model is only compatible with what I shall call for convenience's sake medical equality on wholly unrealistic assumptions as to the percentage of total national wealth to be devoted to health. Certainly it is not expected that a doctor will do the impossible. If a disease is incurable the personal care model does not require a cure. Similarly, if drugs, appliances, or surgical techniques exist in some distant place and the doctor has no means at his disposal to obtain them for his patient, then there too the condition is *pro tanto* incurable. These are obvious points, but they show something about the personal care model. It is no part of that model, I believe, that the doctor should actually sacrifice himself for the sake of his patient. There is no entailment in that model that, for instance, the doctor should at his own expense somehow procure the rare drug from half way round the world to help his patient.[35] Similarly, although there may be occasional emergencies such as epidemics or disasters, it is no part of the personal care model that the doctor in general should work for no compensation, for 18 hours a day. In other words, moving towards a necessary specification of the personal care model under the pressure of reality, we may say that though the doctor must provide the best care for each patient, he need only provide the best care he is able to give, and that ability is not measured simply by the physical limits of endurance.

But what does the ideal of personal care mean for the physician in the British National Health Service with a panel of 3,000 patients and a chronically overcrowded consulting room? If the doctor

---

[34] *The Statistical Abstract of the United States — 1972*, table 97, p. 68, median net earnings of physicians from practice rose from $ 22,000 in 1959 to $ 41,500 in 1970.

[35] See the long quotation from the *Indian Law Commissioners Code*, quoted in note 38 to Chapter 3.

in this situation is not only justified but obligated to do his best
for *all* his patients, do we not then have the equivalent in respect
to the individual doctor of what I have called the optimization
model? For what is the individual physician to do? Surely what
he must do is make something like a cost-benefit analysis, optimizing the resources available to him (primarily his time) relative
to the number and the seriousness of the complaints he is called
upon to treat, and the extent to which the expenditure of his time
will serve to benefit a patient. There may be very serious conditions
about which he can do little or nothing and some far less serious
conditions which he might ameliorate through the expenditure of
greater amounts of effort. Should we come to the conclusion that
the personal care model may in fact be an impossibility in everything but a nonexistent, ideal world, with the result that we find
ourselves with a full-blown version of the social responsibility
model?

If we consider not just the attentions of the doctor but various
things that he might do that cost money this uncomfortable conclusion becomes all the more pressing. Since I do not wish to
move yet into a consideration of the hospital situation, the best
example of this point relates to laboratory tests, X-rays and the
like. There is surely a sense in which a great many of the patients
who come to the doctor with various kinds of nonspecific ailments
might conceivably profit from a rather large battery of expensive
laboratory tests. There are also judgments to be made about
what tests should be ordered for persons with no complaints, but
undergoing routine examination. It is evident that some kind of
cost-benefit calculation, however crude and approximate, is involved in deciding these matters. Not only is the doctor concerned
about the drain on his own time, but he has some concern in
avoiding unnecessary expenses to his patients. And where the costs
are borne by third parties, including private insurers, there are
external constraints on his decision as well. The most important
of these will surely be imposed by the Professional Standards
Review Organizations mandated by the new Title XI of the Social
Security Act to pass on the costs and quality of federally reim-

bursable medical care.[36] Finally, if care is provided in a public or private clinic or in a prepaid medical plan, cost and quality guidelines are usually communicated to the individual doctor. An analogous situation exists in Great Britain under the National Health Service.

What is striking is that although doctors both in the United States and Great Britain have in fact responded to increased demands for their services by what might be termed adjustments in the direction of efficiency, the claim is still generally being made that the care they give their patients corresponds to the personal care model, more or less.[37] Where there are complaints about their ability to render the highest quality service, these complaints tend to refer to inadequate facilities, waiting lists at hospitals, and the like. Individual physicians do not often admit that they themselves are forced to cut corners in the amount of attention they are giving their patients. In this regard the only complaint they make is that they must spend too long hours or that they must deal with their patients in a hurried although, of course, always completely adequate way. Is it really possible that in terms at least of the doctor's own time, the greatly increased effective (effective in the sense that more people now can call on resources) demand on the doctor's time has been met simply by increasing the number of doctors and making them spend longer hours and waste less time? It should be obvious how difficult it would be to obtain anything like reliable data bearing on this point, but some inferences might be hazarded. Although some proportion of doctors will adopt, more or less deliberately, something of an "equipment maintenance scheduling" attitude towards their panel of patients, I would suggest that a significant proportion display a more complex attitude which preserves something of the features of the personal care model.[38]

---

[36] Title XI, Social Security Act of October 30, 1972, 42 U.S.C.A. 1301 et seq. For debates in the American Medical Association regarding this legislation, see N. Y. Times, October 28, 1973, p. 1, col. 3.

[37] See M. Feldstein, *Economic Planning for Health Services Efficiency* (1967), p. 3, 190, Lindsey, supra note 21, Chapters 8 and 9.

[38] See Blumgart, "The Medical Framework for Viewing the Problem of Human Experimentation" in *Daedalus*; Hiatt, "Social Medicine: A Need for Bridges to

The best physicians rarely if ever deliberately cut back from what they consider to be optimum personal attention to each of their patients. They will tell you, they will sincerely believe, and their behavior will at least in part confirm, that with each patient they take just as much time and trouble as that patient's needs require. But with growing demand, of course, something has to give. What happens, I would suggest, is this combination of circumstances: The queues for doctors with this attitude inevitably lengthen, so that even though one gets the full measure of attention when his turn comes, it may take longer and longer for that turn to come. The result must be that this delay in some cases is itself prejudicial to the health of the patient — there may be queues, after all, even of emergency cases. And others are forced to join other queues that may be shorter because the doctor is less sought after or dispenses his care more expeditiously. But I would suppose there are other adjustments as well. Each visit becomes somewhat shorter, somewhat more expeditiously handled, somewhat more streamlined. And this may still be compatible with an attitude and practice which do not dismiss as too remote or "not worthwhile" lines of inquiry that might be pursued, because pursuing them would prejudice others waiting in the queue. This is not to say that even the most conscientious and scrupulous of physicians will not make the judgment that certain possibilities are too far-fetched to be pursued. But these judgments are judgments that would probably be made even if the doctor had all the time in the world; they would be made partly because of the doctor's own self-esteem and partly out of a sense that excessive scrupulosity is not conducive to an appropriate attitude on the part of the patient towards his own health.

The most interesting, elusive, and subtle adaptation to the increased demand would be a more or less unconscious adjustment on the part of the most conscientious, traditional physician in his view of what constitutes that highest level of professional care which he insists on giving to all his patients, no matter how

Other Disciplines" *The Harvard Magazine* (Spring, 1974); Ramsey, *The Patient as Person* (1970).

long a queue for his services results.[39] Just because what consti-tutes this kind of attention will be a matter of judgment, of tradition, of habit and of intuition it is reasonable to suppose that the pressures on all of these subtle factors could bring about gradual shifts in the expectations of patients as to what constitutes ideal attention on the part of their physician. That is to say, neither doctor nor patient will feel that once the patient's turn in the queue does come, the patient is getting anything else but full personal attention, even though the expectations and practice of what constitutes this full personal attention may have in part adjusted to the pressure of increased numbers.

5.2.2. The hospital

When one moves to the level of the hospital the tale becomes easier to tell, because the applicability of the optimization model is far clearer. Those giving service in a hospital are generally under the control and direction of chiefs of service, chief medical officers, or boards of trustees whose responsibility is explicitly a corporate responsibility.[40] These doctors do not have patients in the sense that they administer care in a personal, face-to-face, one-by-one fashion. Their responsibility is to a defined group of patients, and the nurses, interns, residents and others act under the specific direction of what one might call these group doctors. Now the position of the intern or resident who is charged with giving the front-line care in a hospital is consequently rather ambiguous. In

---

[39] An analogous issue obtains in many public defender organizations, where there are chronic shortages of lawyers to handle the cases of the indigent criminal defendants whom they are supposed to service. Some organizations try to help all these defendants, and so feel forced to resort to wholesale guilty pleas with some relief for the client in sentencing. Others insist on inquiring more closely into each case, bringing the case to trial if the client insists, and mounting a full-scale defense. In the latter type of organization there is an inevitable piling up of cases, and the courts are forced to appoint additional counsel or even to dismiss cases where too long a delay results.

[40] See Somers and Somers, supra note 18, at p. 57; W. McNervey, *Hospital and Medical Economics*, vol. 1, Chapter 2 (1962); A. Moss, *Hospital Policy Decisions: Process and Action* (1966).

terms of medical ethics and law he does assume a personal professional obligation to the particular patient when he treats him.
If his standing orders were to give what would be found to be
improper attention, I would assume that like any other subordinate
he would be personally liable for any actions which he knew or
ought to have known were negligent or improper, even though his
actions might also make those on whose orders he acted similarly
liable.

The problem before us, however, rarely if ever involves doing
something actively improper (we will come back to this when we
deal with experimentation specifically) or even anything falling
below a standard which in a court of law or in the proceedings of
a professional society would be found to be unprofessional. Rather
we are concerned with adjusting the level of care and attention
the intern, resident or nurse can give when his time and attention
represent scarce resources in the hospital. At the very least, a
subordinate who consistently gave more care and attention to
fewer patients than the overall staffing needs of the hospital
required would find himself looking for another position. And
where the question is one of ordering tests, surgical procedures
and the like, the directives of group supervisors could hardly be
systematically circumvented.

These inter-relations are illustrated when we consider the norms
for average length of hospital stay in various classes of conditions.
For instance, should hospitalization last for two, three or four
weeks after an acute coronary episode?[41] For the patient of a
private physician it is up to that private physician to determine the
length of stay. For a ward patient or a patient who is in some
sense the patient of the organization hospital norms are likely to
be determinative. Indeed such norms will exert influence on the
private physician, as well, since as a physician with admitting
privileges in the hospital he is under considerable pressure not to
stray too far out of line with the standards set by his colleagues,[42]

---

[41] See Mather et al., "Acute Myocardial Infarction: Home and Hospital Treatment" [1971] *Brit. Med. J.* 3, 334.

[42] Moss, supra note 40, at 200–8; Somers and Somers, supra note 18, at 53–71.

particularly where there are waiting lists for entry into the hospital and a failure to abide by these guidelines would prejudice the chances of other doctors' patients' finding hospital beds. Also various financial intermediaries have referred to such norms in determining what level of hospital charges they would stand ready to assume.[43]

Since those on the front-line of patient care in hospitals are under the control of hospital administrators (even though many doctors will in fact occupy both roles at different times of the day), we should turn to those administrators' principles of choice. Most hospital administrators are severely constrained at least in their choice of goals: The kind of hospital, its geographical area, its mode of financing are usually beyond their control. That is why so much even of the recent literature on hospital administration is concerned with ways of cutting costs, given the system and level of benefits the hospital is bound to offer.[44] There is very little systematic explicit consideration of ways to choose between possible benefits, except perhaps in respect to quite marginal issues. Where such decisions are made it is often in terms of pricing policy: What services and what categories of patients will in effect subsidize what others, how much free care will be offered and to whom, and the like. This does not necessarily suggest simply an unwillingness to face hard choices. Rather it may reflect a partial adherence by hospital administrators to the model of personal care. Like private physicians they continue to hold themselves out as offering their traditional services and the only allocational devices resorted to are queuing (waiting lists) and financial barriers. The effect of these is that when someone does not receive help no one in the hospital is in the position of saying that he cannot help because he does not want to, it is only because he cannot. And as financial barriers are dropped through the intervention of government aid

---

[43] Supra, at 68–71; Egdahl, and Saward, supra note 33.

[44] See, e.g., M. Feldstein, *Economic Analysis for Health Services Efficiency* (1967); M. Feldstein, *The Rising Cost of Hospital Care* (1971); W. McNervey, *Hospital and Medical Economics* (1962); American Association of Hospital Consultants, *Functional Planning of General Hospitals* (Mills, ed. 1969).

and private insurance there are shifts in what constitutes the best possible hospital care. The fact that "good care" has required progressively shorter periods of hospitalization after normal delivery or after acute heart attacks may surely be attributable at least in part to the pressure of rising costs.

At the other extreme, when capital improvement decisions or expansion decisions are called for, something approaching the optimization model is far more explicitly in play.[45] The decision not to undertake a particular kind of service, say heart surgery, is recognized to entail the loss of a certain number of statistical lives, but the justification is that the scarce resources available to the hospital can be better used in other ways. Yet here too the adherence to the model is less than complete, for hospital administrators generally think of themselves as serving a particular, traditionally defined community irrespective of whether other communities receive anything like adequate care. Indeed one might analogize the hospital's attitude towards "its" community to a doctor's obligation to "his" patients. The obligation, once undertaken, is binding, but the assumption of the obligation is itself a far more discretionary, arbitrary matter.

5.2.3. The department of health

The third level is that of governmental planners whose task it is to establish health care budgets in the context of a larger responsibility toward the overall welfare of the population to which their particular governmental unit applies. The Department of Health is not like a large hospital, since the hospital is not part of a bureaucracy which it serves. Moreover, this third level of concern is distinguished from those we have considered so far in its remoteness from the provision of care to identified persons. Perhaps the chief administrator of a large hospital is also very remote, but his colleagues in whose physical presence he works constantly include many who are on the front-lines and so his task maintains

---

[45] See Moss, supra note 40, at 230 ff; *Functional Planning of General Hospitals*, supra.

him in some contact with such first order activities. One might also mention the fact that traditionally chiefs of service and even directors of hospitals have been doctors, and have passed through careers which involved a certain amount of front-line medical care. There is a sense in which they may still look upon the patients in their hospital as *their* patients. It also should be noted that these second order providers, while they are forced to adopt optimizing decision techniques in respect to the patients already in their hospitals, very often recur to waiting lists as an allocational device in determining who shall enter their hospital in the first place. This would suggest that they feel an obligation to do the best by *all* the patients under their actual care in the hospital at any time, but that the intensity of their concern drops rapidly in respect to those who are only potential patients in the hospital. Here again third order decision makers cannot easily make such distinctions.

There may be times when government officials do adopt an attitude that approaches the personal care model. In cases of emergencies, disasters, and calamities government officials may authorize the expenditure of resources in ways quite inconsistent with their avowed overall policies. Some of the reasons for this I have adverted to in Chapter 3. The response might be in fact only apparently irrational; it might be good policy. But there must be another sense in which the sudden calamity dramatizes and thus identifies and individualizes in an unusual way certain members of the general population, that general population which the decision maker is usually concerned with only in a general way. I shall not go into this matter further. It is interesting and difficult, but for the third level of decision it is important only as the extraordinary event. And by hypothesis an extraordinary event must be extraordinary; it cannot be a situation which is confronted every day and the response to it cannot become that response which is the general way of doing business. For the first order decision maker, by contrast, there are nothing but front-line, personalized decisions to be made.

In considering the processes involving the third order decision maker I shall not here review the relatively new but burgeoning

literature in health economics.[46] It is sufficient to point out the
nature of the responsibilities and the inevitably general modes of
analysis and decision employed. It is striking that higher level
governmental officials charged with responsibility for health care
have to date used very little of the armament of decision and
cost-benefit analysis, PPB, and the like. Indeed it seems that the
size of overall health budgets is often determined in haphazard,
accidental and sometimes even whimsical ways. A general goal,
such as the conquest of cancer is set and then an almost arbitrary
price tag is placed on this objective. Or total amounts available
may be determined simply by taking the previous year's figures and
adding a certain percentage as the normal increment.[47]

My conclusion is that the further the government bureaucrat
moves from a rigorous application of the optimizing model, the
more his conduct will be arbitrary, irrational, undesirable. But
since those at the highest levels of the system make decisions
which impinge upon every concrete manifestation of the system,
should this conclusion lead to the further conclusion that, after all,
the optimizing model is and always has been the correct, the
rational model *for agents at all levels of the system*? And if so,
what does this do to the analysis and conclusions of the previous
chapters?

5.3. *The antinomy confronted: putting the two models together*

5.3.1. *The rightness of queuing*

In Chapter 3 I set out the four rubrics under which the rights in

---

[46] See authorities cited in notes 4 to 10 to Chapter 4. For good introductions and
surveys, see Feldstein, "The Medical Economy" 229 *Scientific American* 151 (September, 1973); Ruderman, "Economic Aspects of Health Planning" in *The Theory and
Practice of Public Health* (Hobson, ed., 3rd ed. 1969). Arrow, "Uncertainty and the
Welfare Economics of Medical Care," 53 *Amer. Econ. Rev.* 941 (1963), is an elegant
introduction at a more advanced and abstract level.

[47] See generally Maddox, "Muddling Through: Planning for Health Care in

personal care may be collected: lucidity, autonomy, fidelity and humanity. These are not themselves the rights in the doctor-patient relationship but rather the characteristics which that relationship will manifest when the rights of doctors and patients are respected in it. The relationship is marked by candor, lack of imposition, loyalty to the interests of the patient, and a humane concern for his condition. The whole makes up the concept of personal care. What we must now see is what the meaning of these rights might be in the conditions or relative scarcity I have sketched.

Scarcity impinges on the implementation of these rights in two different ways: (1) Avoiding fraud, violence, or breach of faith or cruelty makes it more costly to benefit others generally — nowhere is this as clear as in the case of experimentation. Our unwillingness to violate a patient's rights may prevent us testing a treatment that will save future persons great suffering. (2) Respecting these rights of one patient may seem to preclude our doing the same for another. If lucidity implies explanation and explanation takes time, then not all may be vouchsafed the full explanation they may need. Or fulfilling the expectations of one patient faithfully may mean violating those of another. Now my thesis holds that the realization of the bond of significant personal relationships takes precedence over the conferring of benefits in abstract, impersonal relations. Benefits conferred in the context of particular, concrete relations are not only weightier *goods* than impersonal benefits but involve *rights*. And these rights must not be compromised, because candor and faithfulness are the very conditions of any significant personal relations at all. To stand ready to compromise them is not to be a little bit impersonal, a little bit unfaithful, somewhat fraudulent and violent. It is to deny the integrity of personal relations altogether; personal relations and the recognition of the rights in them are correlative concepts. And a life without personal relations, where personal relations are sacrificed to the good of the group is like a life where fulfilment is

England" 9 *Medical Care* 439 (1971); M. Feldstein, *Economic Analysis for Health Service Efficiency* (1967), Chapter 1.

continuously postponed to some indefinite future. For it is in the concreteness of personal relations that the coherence and concreteness of our values is rooted. And the rights in personal relations are the constituting principles of personal relations.

I conclude therefore that the rights in personal care must not be sacrificed for what to the primary care provider are abstract persons and abstract goods. This means that the structure of the relationship, its respect for lucidity and the rest must be maintained in the face of the claims of the optimization model. The difficulty with this conclusion appears to come in respect to the second type of conflict where rendering personal care to one man precludes not some abstract, impersonal benefit to a distant person but rather precludes rendering personal care itself to another. There are, to be sure adjustments that the physician can make in the face of the needs of other potential patients. He may spend less time, observe fewer conventional amenities, but past a point the good of personal care is indivisible. The doctor must take the time to learn about and take into account the personal situation, needs and values of his patient — insofar as these may be relevant and implicated in the preservation of health, of bodily and thus of personal integrity in the treatment. If he does not the patient becomes simply a factor in an overall social equation which the doctor serves to optimize. It is the patient's particularity that makes him a person and relevant attention to it that makes personal care.

But what of those who are deprived of care as a result of this indivisibility of personal care?

Since personal care is a personal relation, with personal claims on the part of the patient and a personal obligation on the part of the doctor, personal care will entail the characteristics of personally assumed obligations. For instance, if the minimum requirements of personal care vary and develop as the doctor learns more about his patient, then those developing needs themselves will in part determine the allocation of time and resources to that patient. The surgeon may not put down his knife, as it were, to attend to another patient, just because the first operation ends up taking longer than he had expected — though perhaps he might if the first operation is for the removal of a wart and the second is a life-threatening emergency. To have entered upon care is to create an obligation, a nexus, and the very concept of care requires that this be followed through. An analogy: Perhaps there is some proper allocation of time and energy that a person should make between the interests of his children and those of the larger society. And suppose that a man and a woman have that number of children which reasonably seems to maintain this proper proportion, yet with illness or changed circumstances their children require a vastly greater portion of their time. They must then "follow through." Obligation means that a relation having been entered into, must be seen through.[48] And it is of the essence of the doctor-patient relationship that it is the creation of a relationship and the assuming of an obligation. Yet it is inevitable that this structuring of the social situation in terms of relationships and their obligations will allocate a greater proportion of time to those who are in existing situations of obligation, than to those to whom obligations have not yet been assumed. And the only consolation that can be offered to the latter is that the violence that would have to be done in order to serve their interests would be a violence that ultimately would destroy the world for which they wish to survive.

Is this a satisfactory answer to those who do not receive a share of this indivisible good? I now go on to argue that it is and it is not. In respect to the individual doctor it is a satisfactory answer. He must fulfil the obligations of the situations in which he finds himself. That situation may have come about through chance — he finds himself on the scene of an accident, and will not come away to answer another call on his services. But often the situation

---

[48] For a good survey of the philosophical position that obligations, *first* have a special moral stringency, and *second* that obligations are either entered into or arise out of special, defined relationships between identified persons, see Ladd, "Legal and Moral Obligation" in *Political and Legal Obligation — NOMOS XII* (Pennock and Chapman, ed. 1970); see also Hart, "Legal and Moral Obligation" and Urmson, "Saints and Heroes", both in *Essays in Moral Philosophy* (Melden, ed. 1958); J. Rawls, *A Theory of Justice*, § 52 (1971). Note 32 to Chapter 3 and accompanying text are also relevant to this point.

did not come about through chance at all: There are too few doctors available because adequate plans were not made for physician training. Medicines or hospital beds are not available because resources are devoted to other uses. These decisions may reflect poor judgment, mistaken priorities or unjust diversion of resources on the part of second or third level providers. Yet it is fallacious to argue from the premise that in another, better world where everyone did his duty no one would be without care, to the conclusion that, therefore, I must myself single-handedly try to approximate the conditions of such a world even where others have failed in their obligations. I need not sacrifice myself to right the wrongs of others. All the more so I need not, indeed I must not, violate my obligations to identified others for the same reason.

The point is a deep and pervasive one, and brings up again my running quarrel with utilitarianism and its economic counterparts. A morality of rights and obligations asserts a difference between my being the author of another's harm and that harm coming about through the wrong of a third person, though I might have prevented it. If I failed to prevent it because of a duty to another or because of my concern for my own well-being, I may have acted within my rights. I may indeed have been bound not to violate an undertaking to another. For respect of my autonomy should leave me free — even morally free — to pursue my own concept of the good without the constant imposition that would be entailed by a duty to right the wrongs of third persons to strangers. And if I am entitled so to prefer myself, so long as I do not harm others, surely I may dispose of this same autonomy by freely binding myself to some chosen person, to whom I *must* then grant the same preference that *I may* show to myself. That the good man will so bind himself to others is unquestionable, but if goodness and autonomy are to be compatible, then the subject and extent of my friendship and personal relations should not be determinable by the wrongs of others. I must do what is right for me, even though others may not do what is right for them.

In general, if I have undertaken (perhaps entirely voluntarily) an obligation to certain defined persons, the fact that others have failed in their obligations to other persons neither compels nor justifies my violating my own obligations in order to pick up the slack produced by others. It is on this basis that we regretfully put the lives and well-being of our own family and friends (indeed of ourselves) ahead of equally urgent interests of more remote persons, when the perils and the situation of those other persons have not been brought about by our actions.[49] It is interesting to note that only the classical utilitarian would deny this natural preference, asserting in his rigorously consistent way that it is the obligation of each of us to give equal weight to the interests of all. (Of course the utilitarian will seek to explain our tendency to prefer those to whom we stand in special relationships either in terms of an imperfectly developed moral sense or in terms of the argument that those closest to us just are that class of persons whom in fact we are in the best position most efficiently to assist.)

The picture I offer, therefore, is the picture of the responsible doctor adjusting his time to the length of his queue, cutting out certain features of the care that he gives, pressing himself and his patients, and yet stopping short, digging in his heels and saying that if he had to economize further in the giving of medical care, it would be as if he were giving no care to anybody. So as far as the doctor is concerned, there is a queue for his services. And since it is better that some receive personal care than that none do, and since he is in the relationship that he is to those patients who are already before him, then he must let those at the end of the queue take care of themselves. True, it is not their fault that they are at the end of the queue; but it is not the doctor's fault either.[50]

---

[49] See note 33 to Chapter 3.

[50] Professor Anscombe, in a brief note "Who is Wronged?" 5 *Oxford Review* 16 (1968), makes the following suggestive argument: If I give one patient a massive dose of a drug that could be divided up and used to save five people, not one of those five who might have been saved can claim that *he* has been wronged, that I owed the smaller dose of the drug to *him*. "... Yet all can reproach me if I gave it to none. It was there, ready to supply human need, and human need was not supplied. So any one of them can say: you ought to have used it to help us who needed it; and so all are wronged. But if it was used for someone, as much as he needed it to keep him alive, no one has any ground for accusing me of having wronged *himself*. — Why, just because he was one of five who could have been saved, is he wronged

5.3.2. *The obligations of bureaucrats*

If the fulfilment of their obligations by primary care providers results in disparities between the care received by the rich and the poor or maybe just between the lucky and the unlucky; if queuing is the determinative distributional device, it is the responsibility of those at the secondary and tertiary levels to remove the disparities. For it is their responsibility to provide for the welfare of populations as a whole. As we have seen, the objects of their humanity can only appear to them as groups and abstractions, and indeed any concern for particularity on their part is nothing other than corruption and arbitrariness.

This is not to say that for bureaucrats there are not moral constraints on the pursuit of the greatest good of the greatest number. Their systems must be adequate and efficient but above all they must be just. The systematic, general character of the constraint of distributive justice makes it the ethical consideration specifically directed to those who design and operate systems, while its application grows unclear and anomalous when it is proposed

---

in not being saved, if someone is supplied with it who needed it? What is his claim, except the claim that what was needed go to him rather than be wasted? But it was not wasted. So he was not wronged. So who was wronged? And if no one was wronged, what injury did I do?

"Similarly if there are a lot of people stranded on a rock, and one person on another, and someone goes with a boat to rescue the single one, what cause, so far, have any of the others for complaint? They are not injured unless help that was owing to them was withheld. There was the boat that could have helped them; but it was not left idle; no, it went to save that other one. What is the accusation that each of them can make? What wrong can he claim has been done him? None whatever: unless the preference signalizes some ignoble contempt.

"I do not mean that, because they are more, isn't a good reason for helping these and not that one, or these rather than those. It is a perfectly intelligible reason. But it doesn't follow from that that a man acts badly if he doesn't make it his reason. He acts badly if human need for what is in his power to give doesn't work in him as a reason. He acts badly if he chooses to rescue rich people rather than poor ones, having ill regard for the poor ones because they are poor. But he doesn't act badly if he uses his resources to save X, or X, Y and Z, *for no bad reason*, and is not affected by the consideration that he could save a larger number of people. For, once more: Who can say he is wronged? And if no one is wronged, how does the rescuer commit any wrong?"

for those who confront only particular individuals in discrete cases. Other virtues, other claims predominate at that particular level.

Thus, the issue of fairness, of justice, is of particular concern to the health care bureaucrat. It is his regulations, resource allocation decisions, his incentive structures which will determine the circumstances, the quantity of resources, and the length of the queues when doctors encounter patients and assume obligations to them. It is the task of bureaucrats to define the level of training and the allocation between generalists and specialists.[51] Therefore, it is up to these bureaucrats so to arrange things so that the benefits of primary care are distributed in a fair and equitable way. While I have argued that it is not the responsibility, indeed it is inimical to the responsibility, of the physician to seek to implement some overall notions of fairness in the ways in which he provides care to individuals, it does not at all follow that stringent obligations of this sort do not rest on the higher level bureaucrat. If minimal health care might be regarded as a good which cannot be subdivided past a certain point, so that the attempt to make it smaller and go around to more people would destroy it entirely, this does not at all imply that the overall system should not provide the appropriate amount of this good or distribute it as fairly as possible among the population.

Finally, it is worth making quite explicit a moral assumption of the foregoing argument. I readily concede that everything need not work out for the best in the far from perfect world we have been considering. It is possible that government officials will stupidly or corruptly fail to perform the functions on which the fairness of the outcome of the total system depends. The result will be suffering and privation. Does that show my argument is wrong, that primary care providers should abandon in such cases the obligations of their roles? Why? Who says that it is a test of a sound set of moral principles that pain is reduced in it to a lower

---

[51] See, e.g., Ebert, "The Medical School" 229 *Scientific American* 138 (September, 1973); *Royal Commission on Medical Education Report on Medical Education 1965-1968* (1968).

point than in all competitors? That is not my view. We must
reduce the suffering of men, but not so much because suffering is
bad, as because it is human beings who are suffering. Consequently
it is more important that we retain respect for our own and each
other's humanity as we relieve suffering, than that suffering be
relieved. After all, as I argued in the previous chapter, suffering
like death will always be with us.

CHAPTER 6

The practice of experimentation

The British and Danish randomized clinical trials designed to test the relative efficacy of simple versus radical mastectomy as a therapy for cancer of the breast have already been described at the beginning of Chapter 3. The fact that, so far as the published reports indicate, the women receiving the therapies knew neither that they were participating in an experiment nor that their surgery was being determined at random illustrates the moral dilemmas of such RCT's. In this chapter I will bring to bear the different levels of the preceding theoretical discussion on the uneasy case of the RCT. The case is uneasy because of the strong and plausible claim that the RCT represents the best hope of advancing medicine and so alleviating suffering, but appears to do so only by disregarding the rights of patients. In this Chapter at last I hope to offer specific judgments about what patients' rights in experimentation are, and how some of the current practice of RCT's may violate them. I also plan to consider the social claim — heretofore discussed only generally — that the recognition of these rights may in the context of the RCT be too finicky, too costly, and to conclude just how much cost we should accept in procuring the social benefits of experimentation. Finally, I will offer some practicable suggestions for resolving the conflict between individual rights and the social goals of experimentation in a way that is true to the principles of each. At this point I should recall again a point made in the introduction: I am leaving totally out of account the special problems relating to experiments with children, mentally impaired persons, and others who are permanently or temporarily deprived of the ordinary capacity to understand and choose in a medical situation. Certainly I can see that these present important issues, but I feel justified in abstracting from them because their difficulty comes as much from an understanding of the special status of these groups as it does from problems of experimentation and consent generally.

My analysis will have more concreteness and immediacy if I add to the account of the breast cancer studies mentioned above, brief descriptions of three other well known and influential RCT's which have recently been carried out.

6.1. Some recent randomized clinical trials

6.1.1. The Veterans' Administration cooperative study group: clinical trial of anti-hypertensive therapy

The high incidence of mortality and morbidity associated with hypertension has long been well known. Sufferers from high blood pressure are far more prone among other things to stroke, heart and kidney disease. Certain drugs are known to lower the measured blood pressure, but with serious side effects such as depression, fatigability and impairment of sexual function.[1] To test whether these drugs simply ameliorated the measurable manifestation of hypertension, or whether they reach the underlying conditions which were associated with the danger to life and health, patients at Veterans' Administration clinics in a number of cities were randomized in a double-blind RCT between anti-hypertensive drugs and placebo therapy.[2] Except in the case of

---

[1] Frohlich, "Hypertension 1973: Treatment — Why and How," 78 *Annals of Internal Medicine* 717, at 720 (1973).

[2] Freis, "Organization of a Long Term Multi-Clinic Therapeutic Trial in Hypertension" in *Anti-Hypertensive Therapy: Principles and Practice* (Gross, ed. 1966); Veterans' Administration Cooperative Study Group on Hypertensive Agents "Effects

important untoward events, neither the patient nor his attending physician knew into which group a patient fell; thus the test was double-blind. Mortality and morbidity in the control group of patients with severe hypertension was so much higher, that the trial was discontinued and all the surviving patients in that group placed on the anti-hypertensive drugs. The trial was, however, continued for a further period of years for somewhat less severe cases, but eventually the same conclusion was reached.

Although the published reports of these trials go into considerable detail regarding the devices used to determine whether the participants had in fact been following their regimen, nothing at all is said regarding the nature of the disclosure to the participants and the kind of consent that was obtained.[3]

6.1.2. The university group collaborative oral anti-diabetic agent randomized clinical trial.[4]

The development of agents taken orally to control blood sugar levels in diabetics was and by many doctors and patients still is considered a great boon, doing away with the need for several

---

of Treatment on Morbidity in Hypertension" 213 *J.A.M.A.* 1143 (1970); "Effects of Treatment on Morbidity and Hypertension," 202 *J.A.M.A.* 1028 (1967). These and other Veterans' Administration Cooperative Study Group RCT's are described by Chalmers, and Shaw and Chalmers, notes 10 and 23 to Chapter 3. The Cooperative Study Groups have performed RCT's in respect to the efficacy of anti-coagulants after myocardial infarction and strokes, preventive portacaval shunt surgery, and therapies for carcinoma of the prostate.

[3] Chalmers, and Shaw and Chalmers, supra, in describing Veterans' Administration trials generally, state that informed consent is obtained as a matter of principle, unless the subject would be too disturbed by the disclosure or could not comprehend it. In such cases the consent of a relative is obtained. There is some question about what the disclosure contains. It is not stated that the fact of randomization is disclosed.

[4] See Knattered et al., "Effects of Hypoglycemic Agents on Vascular Complications in Patients with Adult-Onset Diabetes" 217 *J.A.M.A.* 777 (1971); "Sulfonylureas: Effects in Vivo and in Vitro — N.I.H. Conference", 75 *Annals of Internal Medicine* 607 (1971); Schwartz, "The Tolbutamide Controversy: A Personal Perspective" 75 *Annals of Internal Medicine* 303 (1971); "Tolbutamide (Orinase) and Diabetes" *The Medical Letter*, vol. 12, no. 24 (Issue 310) (November 2, 1970).

insulin injections a day. In order to test the efficacy and toxicity of these agents a double-blind randomized trial was mounted in several centers. Early in the trial evidence appeared that not only were the expected benefits not forthcoming, but that there appeared to be a statistically significant increased incidence of cardiovascular disease associated with these drugs. The code was broken, the drugs ceased to be administered and the trial ended. But many complained that this was done at too early a stage, that if more evidence had come in the drugs would have been vindicated;[5] yet those responsible for the trial could not in conscience continue in the face of the early unfavorable evidence. As a consequence some consider the results inconclusive and the drug continues in general use to this day by many but not all practitioners.

6.1.3. Coronary by-pass surgery[6]

In recent years techniques have been developed for by-passing regions of serious atherosclerotic blockage in the major coronary arteries, and thus permitting increased blood supply to the heart muscle below these blockages. There have, however, been serious questions raised regarding the efficacy of this technique in certain cases of coronary artery disease, and some responsible persons have questioned whether in certain situations the more traditional "best" therapies and regimens might not be as good if not better.[7] Moreover, the incidence of surgical mortality itself is far from negligible, and the operation is extremely costly in terms of time, technical resources and blood needed for transfusion. If the claims of the more enthusiastic proponents of this technique were

---

[5] Gubner, "Treatment of Diabetes: Effect on Cardiovascular Disease" *Medical Tribune* (September 7, 1970).

[6] See, e.g., Auer et al., "Direct Coronary Artery Surgery for Impending Myocardial Infarction" 44 *Circulation* 102 (1971); Cohn et al., "Aorto-coronary by-pass for acute coronary occlusion" 64 *J. Thoracic and Cardiovascular Surgery* 503 (1972); Gorbin, "Indications for Surgery in Patients with Coronary Heart Disease" vol. 3, no. 2 *Cardiac Surgery* 1, 72.

[7] Editorial, *The Lancet* 137 (January 20, 1973).

valid[8] there would be many hundreds of thousands of good candidates for this surgery each year at staggering social cost.

In order to evaluate the claims for coronary by-pass surgery in various categories of disease, a number of hospitals throughout the country have instituted randomized clinical trials.[9] In one trial, participants are referred by their physician to cardiologists in the participating hospital. The participants are told that a study is being conducted in which they are involved, that they will receive the best available treatment for their case, and that they are free not to join in or stay in the study. Although they know of the alternative therapies, only if they ask are they told that the choice is determined by a randomizing scheme.

6.1.4. The Salk polio vaccine trial

The Salk vaccine was the first effective preventive measure against poliomyelitis. It was originally introduced in a nation-wide, double-blind, randomized, placebo controlled trial in which hundreds of thousands of children were entered by their parents. The fullest disclosure of the risks and potential benefits was made, and the mechanism of the trial was also fully disclosed. The vaccine was not available outside of the trial. Parents were told that if the trial was successful the control group and the families of all participants would have first call on the vaccine thereafter.[10]

In Chapter 3 I reviewed briefly the ways in which the RCT does in fact impose burdens on the individual participants in each particular case, even though perhaps the overall result might be a great social good, a social good indeed in which these or other individual patients might subsequently participate. In this section I shall consider more fully and precisely the ways in which

---

[8] Sheldon et al., "Vein Graft Surgery for Coronary Artery Disease" *Circulation*, Supplement III to vol. 47–48, p. 184 (1973).

[9] See, e.g., Hultgren et al., "Veterans' Administration Study of Coronary By-passes" 289 *N. Engl. J. Med.* 105 (July 12, 1973).

[10] See T. Francis et al., *Evaluation of the 1954 Field Trial of Poliomyelitis Vaccine* (1957); Zeisel, in *Annals*, at 483 n. 8.

the RCT might violate the system of rights I have been elaborating.

The obvious intuitive objections to the RCT are two: *First*, the protocol may require an abdication of professional judgment such that the patient's therapy is determined not by the needs of his particular case but by the demands of the experimental design. *Second*, the practice of RCT's often, though not necessarily, involves deceit. The patient believes that his doctor is determining his therapy solely on one basis, while there are other factors involved about which the patient is not informed, and which might lead him to withdraw from the care of that particular doctor if he knew of them. A separate, subsidiary objection arises in those RCT's where the results of the trial are not communicated to the patient or even to his doctor until some predetermined stopping point, some predetermined level of significance is attained. The developing results are held in escrow, as it were, by a supervisory panel, which decides when to release them to doctors and their patients. This device is adopted in order to protect the integrity of the trial from the skewing that would result if patients withdrew or refused to enter on the basis of early, preliminary findings.[11]

The incomplete or deceptive disclosure violates the rights collected under the notion of lucidity, while the determination of treatment (either initially or as information subsequently develops) by criteria other than the particular interests of the particular patient violates rights to autonomy and fidelity. Again the intuitive idea is that the doctor-experimenter does not allow the patient to choose between alternative therapies on one hand, and he deprives the patient of the benefit of his individual professional judgment in choosing the therapy on the other. The idea of personal care, with its demand for undivided loyalty to the interests of the patient would thus seem to be violated by this abdication of professional judgment in the interests of the experiment, interests which are not the same as those of the patient in the particular case.

Nor is this even a case where conferring personal care on one

[11] See Chalmers, note 10 to Chapter 3. The issue was important in the diabetes study discussed above. See also the discussion in Chapter 2, § 2 d and e.

patient means depriving another of that care; personal care is abrogated for generalized, social purposes.

6.2. The concept of professional knowledge

The realities of medical practice and the sociology of scientific truth suggests that what goes on in the RCT may not be so drastic a violation of rights as first appears. Even where the doctor loyally seeks to do his "best" for the particular patient his understanding of what that best might be is strongly and properly determined by professional standards and criteria. For when it is said the doctor must do his best, this can only mean his best relative to what he knows about the patient's condition and available therapies. That this knowledge is incomplete and probabilistic is obvious. What is less obvious is the social or, more precisely, the professional nature of that knowledge. And the professional nature of medical knowledge has a close relation to the role of medical experimentation in medical practice.

The professional context serves not only to transmit knowledge from one person to another but also to validate what will count as knowledge. The institutional nature of medical knowledge suggests an important general qualification of the decision-theoretic account of rational decision under uncertainty.

The doctor is not alone with his decision for the patient — whatever the doctor's estimate of the probabilities, he must make a decision which is and will be acceptable to his patient, the patient's family and his professional associates. And the patient too does not choose like a Bayesian gambler confronted by lottery tickets and urns filled with different colored balls. The professional relationship affects what he will find acceptable. Now to be sure, all of these complexities can be recast in terms of confidence levels and the like, but this would ignore the institutional structures that control more or less systematically what those confidence levels will be. In short, the decision-theoretic account of medical knowledge — either from the doctor's or the patient's point of view

— is of limited value. It states the conclusion of the process by which confidence is attained, without illuminating the workings of that process.

The distinctive feature of medical knowledge as professional knowledge is its insistence on professional, impersonal (or transpersonal) validation.[12] The myth of the "great doctor" who plays a brilliant hunch performing a miraculous cure where the body of ordinary plodders failed is a persistent myth[13] but bears about as much relation to reality as does the myth of the great courtroom lawyer who by brilliant cross-examination breaks down his client's wicked accuser, forcing him to admit that after all it was he who did it. In reality, the player of unvalidated hunches is more likely to be a charlatan or quack. That is not to say that this myth does not have a powerful hold on the popular imagination, a hold strengthened by the desperation induced by incurable illness or just the normal process of aging.[14]

For all these reasons, the conception of what is good medicine is the product of a professional consensus. As with all procedurally validated truths, however, there is always the possibility that in particular cases the system will turn down a valid, maybe even a crucially valid, hypothesis. But if the institutions are well designed, the costs of this will be far outweighed by the suppression of dangerous quackery and promulgation of sound and helpful therapies.

---

[12] See the quotation from Chalmers, note 10 to Chapter 3, and Shaw and Chalmers, note 23 to Chapter 3. See generally, Parsons, "Research and the Professional Complex" in *Daedalus*; and materials collected in J. Katz, *Experimentation with Human Beings* (1972), pp. 198–235.

[13] See Moore, "Ethical Boundaries in Initial Clinical Trials" in *Daedalus*.

[14] In the exact sciences this socializing process is also present, but with some differences. There is no need to vault over many missing steps of theory and data to arrive at an urgent conclusion. And if the work of a theoretical physicist is unconvincing to his colleagues, the principal consequences relate to the fate of that work and to the future direction of inquiry. See generally T. Kuhn, *The Structure of Scientific Revolutions* (1962). The quack harms those on whom he practices, and if his cures go wrong, he may be held as a criminal. Also, there is not in pure science the temptation to prey on the lucrative desperation of others, with a corresponding need for institutional structure to control that temptation.

This procedural, professional aspect of medical knowledge first of all suggests some qualification (or at least specification) of the personal care model. It is not the case that the physician should do his best for his patient so much as that he should do the best that good medicine prescribes. In a sense, the individual is sacrificed to an overall better outcome, in that what doctor and patient choose is not the untrammelled expression of the knowledge and values of each. It is limited by the professional norms that constrain the doctor's judgment and constrain it in the name of good medicine generally.[15] This constraint, however, reaches so intimately into what the doctor believes and practices that he does not think of himself as sacrificing anything of value in restraining his impulse to try out some desperate guess. On the contrary, he believes that to do otherwise would be to risk harming his patient, and he does not think of himself as helping his patient *as a doctor* if he does otherwise. This is not where the paradox of professional knowledge arises.

The paradox arises just in respect to experimentation — on sick subjects in the course of their treatment — and just in those cases where the RCT is called upon to validate medical knowledge. As medicine has become more and more closely allied with science, as the scientific, that is, the biological and chemical bases of medicine have become better established, good medicine has come to be viewed as in some way related to good science. The sound hypothesis is the scientifically validated one, and as medical hypotheses inevitably relate to many-factored processes for which a complete theoretical account is lacking, good science and, therefore, good medicine are more and more seen as requiring a solid statistical validation.[16] Yet the very concept of good medicine

---

[15] A similar point holds as to the lawyer's duty of loyalty. The lawyer is not entitled to do *whatever* serves his client's interests, but only what is consistent with his position as an officer of the court. This often implies severe constraints.

[16] See A. Cochrane, *Effectiveness and Efficiency* (1972); Chalmers, and Shaw and Chalmers, supra note 12; Rutstein, "The Ethical Design of Human Experimentation" in *Daedalus*; Strauss, letter in 288 *New Engl. J. Med.* 1183 (1973) to the effect that journals should not even publish reports of studies which are so statistically and scientifically flawed that valid conclusions cannot be drawn from them.

precludes the carrying out of the experiment until after the validation: The brilliant hunch is surely not enough to justify the
departure the experiment entails.

The paradox, moreover, has a third branch: Many therapies
accepted as standard, as good medicine on the basis of an older,
statistically less sophisticated empiricism, now become suspect in
the light not just of new knowledge but of new standards of validation.[17] Thus what good medicine requires may sometimes be a
choice among three unacceptable alternatives: nothing; an older,
dubious remedy; and a newer, unvalidated remedy. And even
the prescribed method of validation is not itself medically acceptable in its execution. This is not to say that the situation was better
at an earlier date. On the contrary, it was almost certainly far
worse, far more arbitrary. Not only were therapies accepted on
the basis of inadequate evidence, but the process of experimentation itself more haphazard, brutal and high-handed.[18]

6.3. *Rights in experimentation*

6.3.1. *Lucidity and the duty of candor*

The concept of professional knowledge might be seen as a justification for the frequently incomplete disclosures made in RCT's.
As I indicated in Chapter 2, even the most solicitous of the regulations of experimentation, the NIH regulations, do not clearly
require that the patient be told that his therapy has been chosen
on a randomized basis. It may well be that the coronary by-pass
RCT disclosure which reveals the fact that the relative merits of
the two therapies are being studied, but states that the patient
will receive that therapy which is thought best for his case, is a
sufficient revelation under these regulations. The somewhat strained

---

[17] See Cochrane, supra. He suggests as one example that the Pap smear test for
cervical cancer may prove an overall needless procedure if subjected to an RCT.

[18] *Katz*, at 284–292, gives extensive and chilling accounts of brutal, unconsented
to experimentation prior to the Nazi era.

contention that in each of the RCT's summarized above the choice between the two therapies was in equipoise becomes considerably more plausible when viewed in conjunction with the concept of professional knowledge. One or the other of the two therapies may not seem quite equally eligible to the patient's doctor, but then as a good professional he would demur, saying that *professionally* he had no basis for preferring one to the other, and thus was justified in viewing them as being in equipoise. Yet even this most subtle — perhaps excessively subtle — line of argumentation does not justify less than complete candor, less than complete disclosure of the precise nature of the experiment. Let us make the assumption — often a strained one — that professional judgment is truly in equipoise, and that this condition of indeterminacy has not itself been brought about by so limiting the range of inquiry into the patient's medical condition that factors favoring one or the other of the therapies have simply not been inquired into and thus are not known to exist. There are still two sufficient reasons for insisting on candor and full disclosure. Both refer to the concept of lucidity and the rights implicated in it.

Even in medically equivalent cases, patients may have quite different value systems; their life plans may have quite different structures. And though the overall prognosis, the overall expected value of the two therapies may be practically the same, the composition of the risks and benefits of each therapy might be different. Thus, for instance, surgery for heart disease in some cases might involve a very high initial risk of surgical mortality followed by a very good risk for, say, five years of survival after the surgery, while the standard medical treatment for the same condition might have the same overall mortality expectation, but with a risk of death distributed much more evenly over the period of years. Different people might quite rationally have different preferences about this. Thetis was allowed to choose for her son, Achilles, between a long and undistinguished life and a short life as a hero. Similarly, one life plan might prefer a heavy initial risk with considerable safety thereafter if things go well, while another would prefer to have the risk more evenly spread over the relevant time period. If it is one of the rights of humanity to determine one's own life plan, then surely questions of the distribution of risk over that life plan are crucial variables regarding which a person should be entitled to reflect and make a choice. Less dramatically also, as in the case of the antihypertensive drug trials, side effects such as depression and decreased vitality may have different significance for different persons. The concept of lucidity, which expresses a fundamental attribute of personality, thus demands a right to confront such information and to choose.

Second, making the even more tenuous assumption now that the therapies are in equipoise even in respect to any matter that could be of relevance to different life plans, failure to disclose deprives the patient of the opportunity to participate intelligently in the processes of his illness and his cure, and thus to make of them significant passages in his life. That the trial will produce information helpful to others supports rather than detracts from the argument. The concept of autonomy, as I have sketched it in Chapter 4, implies a value in being able to control one's own resources, in being one's own man, this value providing the starting point from which generosity, sacrifice and service to others may proceed and assume their full significance. But if participation in an RCT is a form of service, then less than complete disclosure deprives a person of the opportunity of consciously and deliberately rendering service in a crucial social enterprise. This deprivation is aggravated by the fact that those who perpetrate it thereby arrogate all to themselves the opportunity of playing this complex, essential and satisfying social role. Perhaps they fear that if they took their patients as partners, the patients might balk, or might alter the nature of the enterprise. But partnership and trust always entail risks, and always imply a subtle difference in the enterprise pursued in partnership.

6.3.2. *Autonomy and the concept of professional accountability*

The argument that knowledge is professional, and thus a posture of doubt between two therapies is justified, does not for a further reason justify less than full disclosure. The point can be made generally as follows: Candor is required to maintain the integrity of the encounter between physicians and patients as classes, to prevent one from exploiting or subordinating the other to its purposes, and thus to respect the autonomy of both.

More specifically medical truth is professionally validated truth because of the need to protect the class of patients from the ignorance, or enthusiasms, or excesses, or greed of practitioners. But a profession can easily degenerate into a cartel sticking together for mutual protection and profit. Full candor and openness to scrutiny are necessary to ensure that the institutional processes of the profession will serve the client and not the practitioners. Any program of systematic deception, of withholding information that the clients would consider relevant, must be corrupting. In the end the information always gets out anyway, leading to distrust and hostility — a hostility which is likely to be deeper because the client is well aware of his dependence on the profession.[19] And then a group that systematically practices deception on those outside it for some supposedly limited purpose, will tend to lose a sense of responsibility to truth and a respect for those on whom the deception is practiced, both of which are indispensable if the notion of professionally validated truth is to be beneficial and not a cover for mediocrity and self-dealing. These are, to be sure, instrumental considerations, but they are also considerations of principle, considerations of rights. Honesty, candor and thus the protection of the integrity of the relation of doctors and patients are not recommended because of the greater efficiency that obtains when there is integrity. On the contrary, the integrity of that relationship, which recognizes the equal autonomy of both parties to it, is the condition for a kind of cooperation which is often, though not necessarily stable and productive.

---

[19] See generally, DHEW, *Medical Malpractice — Report of the Secretary's Commission on Medical Malpractice* (1973); Glass, "Restructuring Informed Consent — Legal Therapy for the Doctor-Patient Relationship" 79 *Yale L. J.* 1533 (1970).

6.3.3. *Fidelity and humanity*

The imperatives of fidelity and humanity imply rights and duties that further confirm the need for full, effective candor in experimentation. But they go further. They are not satisfied if the patient knows how he is being used, but is given no choice as to his treatment. I have argued in Chapter 4 that a man has a right when he is confronted by another in a concrete situation to demand that his particular situation be taken into account. It is an offense against his humanity to look through his concreteness and see in him only a statistic, only a representative man. And so the professional who undertakes to deal with a patient's serious illness by that undertaking is obligated not only to acknowledge but to respect, to make provisions for the peculiarities, the needs and values of that individual. As I indicated in the previous chapter, the doctor may be severely limited in the resources he has available to him to discharge this obligation, but that is not his fault. The right is fully recognized if the doctor does all that he can. And that is because the recognition of the right is not a matter of achieving this or that ultimate result, but of the parties to the relationship respecting so far as they can the terms of that relationship. Thus to leave the patient no choice but to be a subject in the RCT (however fully disclosed) is inhuman insofar as the physician deliberately withholds from the patient not *information* this time but a treatment which that patient reasonably desires and which it is within the power of the physician to give.

Little more need be said to show how such a proceeding violates the imperatives of fidelity as well. The very vulnerability of the patient to his doctor creates expectations, expectations not just of truthfulness but of humane treatment. To disappoint those expectations is a wrong that goes beyond the actual harm that is done. For in disappointing those expectations the possibility of a system of trust is itself undermined.

6.4. Rights in experimentation: implementation and accommodations

The system of rights in personal care, applied to experimentation, entails the right to full disclosure, to complete candor, and the right not to be experimented upon against one's will, the right to choose one's own therapy with full awareness of the alternatives. But I have acknowledged from the outset of my discussion of rights generally, that rights have limits, that rights conflict, so that those limits must be drawn and accommodations found. If the rights in experimentation I have just mentioned were to spell the end of all experimentation, were to make RCT's and other kinds of experiments impossible, the cost would be enormous. We would have to think again. The picture which the proponents of clinical trials offer is the one in which individuals, choosing rationally in their own self-interest one by one, have collectively chosen a disaster which engulfs them all.[20] In this section I shall argue that this calamitous picture of the consequences of respecting personal care in experimentation is wildly overdrawn. *First,* I shall argue that the costs themselves may have been exaggerated. *Second,* I seek to show that the rights which I affirm are compatible with systems of experimentation that would permit a significant amount of experimentation, including RCT's to go forward. It has not been my argument that there is a personal right to receive medical attention without being involved in experimentation under any and all circumstances, but rather that there are rights *in* personal care which significantly constrain the ways in which experimentation may go forward. But if those constraints are respected there may well be situations in which individuals have little choice but to be part of an experimental study.

6.4.1. Alternatives to randomized controlled trials

Throughout this essay I have concentrated on the nature and

---

[20] For a theoretical account of this phenomenon of collective irrationality, with examples from many fields, see M. Olson, *The Logic of Collective Action* (1965).

problems of the RCT. I have done so because of the recent proliferation of emphatic claims that the RCT is the best, indeed the only scientific way of validating new or old therapies. I have said enough to show that I agree that the RCT has many virtues. In this section I wish to argue quite vigorously that in spite of these virtues the claims for the RCT have been greatly, indeed preposterously overstated. The truth of the matter is that the RCT is one of many ways of generating information, of validating hypotheses.[21] The proponents of the RCT, however, have elevated what is in theory a frequent (though by no means universal) advantage of degree into a gulf as sharp as that between the kosher and the non-kosher.

Inferences drawn from basic scientific theories regarding biologic and chemical processes can and do provide evidence supporting the efficacy of medical therapy. The reason that such theoretical knowledge is rarely sufficient relates to the great gaps in our knowledge and the enormous complexity of the processes in which we intervene. It is just because we often do not know what the biologic and chemical processes are that we must substitute statistical truth for theoretical truth.

Even where the basic science of the processes involved is beyond our reach, the greater our confidence that we have identified all the relevant variables, the less sense it makes to randomize. Let us assume that we are quite sure that age, weight, and sex are the only variables that might affect the efficacy of a drug we are studying, and that we have a model of that effect. Let us further assume that we are quite confident of our ability to measure and define precisely the amounts of the drug administered, its rate of absorption, and the therapeutic and counter-therapeutic effects we are concerned with. In such a case randomization would be a costly and useless refinement. For the only purpose of randomization is to produce confidence in ourselves or others that variables we have not thought of, which we have not controlled for, are

---

[21] For a general introduction, see the articles by Cochrane and Campbell on experimental and quasi-experimental design in *Int. Encyc. Soc. Sci.*, vol. V, at 245. See also *The Quantitative Analysis of Social Problems* (E. Tufte, ed., 1970).

not the crucial variables distorting or producing our results. Indeed when we are sure about our ability to identify and measure the crucial variables, the cheapest, the least intrusive thing to do might be simply to collect data on what others have done in the past, analyzing that data in such a way as to factor out the efficacy of the various elements obtained.

It will be said, quite properly, that we can never know that we have identified and, therefore, can never control for all the crucial variables; also that the identification of these variables may sometimes be more costly and laborious than their statistical elimination through the device of the RCT. I agree that we can never be *sure* that we have identified and controlled for all the crucial variables. But it is ironical that those who, in proposing RCT's defend the concept of statistical truth, fail utterly to recognize that statistical truth is always a matter of degree, that certainty is unavailable anywhere in this life. What counts is the degree of certainty, and in this respect as every other you get what you pay for. Thus the difference between the RCT and the observational, retrospective study is not the difference between good and bad science, truth and falsity, but a difference between varying degrees of confidence. That being the case, the question can *never* be should we accept good or bad science, but is the extra measure of certainty that an RCT might give us in a particular case worth the price. It is ironical indeed that those who, in arguing the need for RCT's, say we must purge ourselves of absolutist thinking regarding the rights of individual patients, engage in absolutist thinking themselves regarding the superiority of randomization. Those who urge an absolutist attitude toward patients' rights may be silly, but they cannot be shown to be wrong according to their own premises. Those who urge an absolute superiority for randomization, by contrast, are making an argument that their own intellectual discipline contradicts.[22] The point is, of course, that

---

[22] I am, I admit, taking the Bayesian side in the controversy between objectivist and subjectivist on Bayesian theories of statistical inference. The objectivist school believes that statistical truth and probability distributions are "out there" and it is the scientist's job to discover them. Although I believe that events and objects are

the campaign for the RCT is waged not in intellectual terms, but in political terms, the enemy being the indolence, self-interest and perhaps even corruption in many sectors of the health care industry and the health care profession. That such indolence, ignorance and corruption exist I would not deny. That it draws around itself the moral mantle of some of the very values I have been arguing for in this essay, I regret. But as intelligent men, let us not be taken in by our own propaganda.

In the balance of this section I will consider ways in which the goals of experimentation might be realized while respecting the rights of individuals in personal care. Many accommodations are in fact possible because the rights I have presented do not in themselves preclude either experimentation or RCT's. But in implementing and accommodating these conflicting considerations we should not proceed on the fallacious assumption that where there is no randomization there is no truth.

6.4.2. *Accommodation by differentiation of role*

The researcher or scientist-doctor who deals directly with patient-subjects may occupy a number of roles. He may be concerned with direct patient care, but he necessarily occupies a role governed by the social responsibility model, since the very purpose of his undertaking is to benefit the general class of patients. The dangers of this dual role have been frequently noted. This dual role might be seen as an attempt to act on both the personal care and the optimization models at the same time. That is why it would be

---

indeed "out there" I hold with the subjectivists that probability and statistics have to do with the practicalities of making the best of a bad job, that is the practicalities of making rational decisions when we cannot know what is out there. For a collection of some basic documents on the subjectivist view, see *Studies in Subjective Probability* (H. Kyburg and Smokler, eds., 1963). An applied text is J.W. Pratt, Raiffa and Schlaifer, *Introduction to Statistical Decision Theory* (1965).

For an example of these disputes in another, controversial area, measuring the efficacy of compensatory education, see Campbell and Erlebacher, "How Regression Artifacts in Quasi-Experimental Evaluation can Mistakenly Make Compensatory Education Look Harmful", in *The Disadvantaged Child*, vol. 3 (Hellmuth, ed., 1970), excerpted in Katz.

far better if in each case the patient's physician were not engaged in experimentation involving that patient at all.[23] Indeed in other professions this conclusion would seem self-evident. As I point out in detail in Chapter 2, an attorney, for instance, could not possibly occupy such a dual role without his client's express consent. Whether or not the duality of role creates a genuine conflict of interest is beside the point. So long as the client might believe there was such a conflict, a full disclosure is required. Nothing justifies a less exigent conception of professional, fiduciary responsibility in the case of the doctor. On the contrary, the whole thrust of my argument has been to establish the rationality of this conception of responsibility to the person.

The second or third level health care provider, by contrast, has no clients, no patients, no responsibility for personal care as such. His concerns are governed and defined by the goals of social responsibility, of distributive justice and efficiency. As to personal care, his responsibility is limited to doing nothing that would compel or induce primary care providers to violate their patients' rights in personal care. In allocating scarce resources it is the administrator's and bureaucrat's job to develop more efficient and effective means of treatment and to evaluate the efficiency and efficacy of existing means.[24]

I should like to explore in regard to experimentation the relation between this obligation at the second and third levels and the constraints and imperatives on the provider of primary care. Consider again the example of research on coronary artery disease therapies. There are two schools of thought about the utility of surgery in certain cases of such disease. Both represent professionally accepted, responsible opinion, and each represents a serious criticism of the other. Intuitively we feel no objection to

---

[23] The point has been made by a number of authors, e.g., Freund, "Introduction" to *Daedalus*; materials collected in *Katz* at pp. 923, 991 and 998; P. Ramsey, *The Patient as Person*, pp. 36, 222, 228 (1970).

[24] A. L. Cochrane, formerly a clinician and now a high official of the British NHS makes a strong statement of his sense that these are his present responsibilities. *Effectiveness and Efficiency*, p. 66 (1972).

second and third order deciders' allowing each school to pursue its cause, subject only to the requirement that detailed records be kept, so that a retrospective analysis can be made to determine the better therapy.[25] Nor do we object to the expenditures of significant resources on the collection and analysis of such data. Such a program on the part of bureaucrats is acceptable because at each level the obligations of that level are being carried out with full respect for the constraints of morality. Certainly there can be no objection to the physicians' supplying data that may allow a definitive conclusion that one or the other of their methods is superior. After all, their loyalty is to their patient's health and to medical knowledge, not to their particular "school", as if it were a religious sect.

There is also no infringement of rights if one "school" receives the same resources as another. It is indeed just an entailment of the notion of professionalism that two alternative theories may attain the status of respectability. So long as both views are responsible and supported by data, the fact that the bureaucracy gives equal support to both is natural. This being so, there is also no problem that the bureaucracy has what might be called a motive of its own in allowing both to go forward: to establish if possible which is best. What is striking is only that this is proper for second and third level providers while such a deliberate failure to choose on the part of the primary care physician raises serious problems. That is because the physician dealing with individual patients must use his personal judgment within the constraints of professionalism, and his refusal to do so is a deliberate withholding of personal attention. To be sure there may not be sufficient scientific grounds for such a preference, and then, as I have argued above, for the doctor to assert a preference may itself be irresponsible. But when there are two schools of thought this means that the professional process has reached not an indeterminate but a double verdict; it is not as if doctors thought the choice were indeterminate, but rather

---

[25] Kaae and Johansen's study of the relative success of more or less radical surgery in cases of breast cancer, discussed in Chapter 3, might be taken as an example of this approach.

that some have reached one, some another verdict, each being prepared to recognize the professional reasonableness of the other. My suggestion would allow administrators at one or two removes to arbitrate between these judgments.

Finally, second and third level providers may be able to use the fact of scarcity and the need to allocate resources fairly and efficiently as the occasion for experimentation, including randomized, controlled experiments. No rights are violated if they reduce subsidies to one kind of therapy (or to the treatment of other conditions) in order to gather and analyze data comparing two therapies. The sums to be allocated to any particular malady cannot be unlimited; the bureaucrat has an obligation to future as well as present sufferers; and thus it follows that there can be no objection to allocations to research as such. This conclusion, so obvious in the context of a retrospective study to decide between two current therapies, is highly suggestive for the issue of the RCT. Coronary by-pass surgery to alleviate certain forms of angina pectoris is obviously ripe for definitive evaluation. And given the large number of factors possibly involved in heart disease, it seems a particular apt case for an RCT. Yet it is also a case in which confidence and candor are crucial. As I have argued, withholding the information that randomization is involved is morally and perhaps legally unacceptable. An experiment relying on withholding the information is deceitful, even if the doctor honestly believes that the choice is so closely balanced as to make the information irrelevant.

Perhaps the dilemma might be avoided by moving to the next level of abstraction. Second and third level providers are far more justified in adopting an attitude of indeterminacy. It is not their job to come to hard but decisive conclusions in particular cases. Moreover, they, unlike individual doctors, are obliged to count the costs of the procedure to the medical system and social system as a whole. Thus it is perfectly acceptable for them to say that in the present state of knowledge only a given percentage of the theoretically eligible persons will be given the operation. It is entirely reasonable to be sparing in the budgetary allocation for an operation that is so much more expensive than an alternative therapy that is judged by some to be just as good. Indeed, the bureaucracy might reasonably decide that any allocation at all to this expensive therapy is acceptable only if the expenditure will also help resolve the doubts.

This leaves the question of fairness in distributing this (somewhat dubious) benefit among those wishing it. Relative urgency of need or capacity to benefit are criteria that have been suggested and indeed used in other cases of scarcity, most dramatically in renal dialysis. But except for categories so gross that they do not accomplish enough, this criterion has properly been criticized as requiring a kind of discrimination and subjectivism that can hardly be defended when one person decides the fate of another.[26] Queuing is far more acceptable since the happenstance of timing at least does not involve one person in choosing among others by highly vulnerable and imprecise criteria. But then a lottery, the device most open to chance, is an even clearer attempt to distribute the benefit in a way that seems fair, at least *ex ante*. Thus the very randomization that achieves fairness may lead to the most accurate evaluation of the effectiveness of this costly and dangerous surgical technique.[27]

It is not now the individual cardiologist who randomizes his patients for the sake of his experiment. Rather the individual cardiologist makes his own independent best judgment for his patient, and then tries to procure the operation for his patient (if that is his decision) in much the same way that he would put his patient on a waiting list for a hospital bed or a kidney transplant. Those chosen would be chosen by a random device. There would

---

[26] For the proposition that lotteries or other randomizing devices represent a fair way of distributing scarce medical resources, see Freund, "Introduction" to *Daedalus*; Katz, "Process Design For Selection of Hemodialysis and Organ Transplant Recipients" 22 *Buffalo L. Rev.* 373 (1973); Sanders and Dukeminier, "Medical Advance and Legal Lag: Hemodialysis and Kidney Transplantation" 15 *U.C.L.A. L. Rev.* 267 (1968); Note, "Scarce Medical Resources" 69 *Colum. L. Rev.* 620 (1969); Ramsey, supra note 23, at pp. 252–59.

[27] Rutstein, supra note 16, also makes the point that randomization might be resorted to for the dual purpose of fairly distributing a desirable scarce resource and most effectively evaluating the efficacy of the particular treatment. The RCT evaluating the Salk Polio vaccine may also have had these characteristics.

be no need for lack of candor anywhere down the line, and the confidence of the patient in his doctor would not be undermined. After all, the doctor holds himself out as a medical expert not a political fixer who can leapfrog the equally good claims of other patients on the list.

6.4.3. Compensation and participation

Relying on scarcity as a device to justify randomization works well only where a number of factors come together. The problem is far harder where one procedure is perhaps promising but truly experimental: where at the moment there is not enough evidence to allow a prudent doctor to say that it is the preferable therapy.[28] Yet with more experience it might turn out clearly so. Or as between two therapies, each championed by its "school" of proponents, no choice can be made on grounds of expense, so that the need to limit the expenditure of scarce medicines cannot come in to justify allocation to one or another therapy by a fair randomizing device. In these and other cases it must be recognized that if experimentation is to take place it must take place as such with the avowal and concurrence of all. But to the extent that patients will not consent, the experiment will not happen, and in the long run the class of patients as a whole will be deprived of beneficial therapies.

In these cases medicine is now more and more forced to rely on volunteers, usually paid volunteers in prisons,[29] or on therapeutic research carried out on desperate cases where a risky, untried procedure offers the only hope.[30] This is an unsatis-

---

[28] As examples of this consider heart transplants and at least the early experience with kidney transplants. For general discussion see Chalmers, "When Should Randomization Begin?" *The Lancet* 858 (April 20, 1968); Moore, "Therapeutic Innovation — Ethical Boundaries in the Initial Trial of New Drugs and Surgical Procedures" in *Daedalus*; and see generally Fox, *Experiment Perilous* (1959) which is excerpted in Katz.

[29] See Zeisel, supra note 10; Katz, "Experimentation With Captive Subjects", Chapter 13, for a collection of materials dealing with this matter.

[30] See Jonas, infra note 32; Moore, supra note 28 and Ramsey, note 1 to Chapter 1, Chapters 1 and 6.

factory situation. The latter expedient cannot be sufficiently widely applicable. And many factors are making the paid volunteer less available. The most important of these is the increased stringency of the requirement of full disclosure of risks. Questions are being raised too about the appropriateness of exploiting any person's peculiar need for money in order to subject him to intimate and often undetermined risks. Reliance on prisoners is problematic for analogous reasons. It is society that has created the situation that makes risking passive mutilation seem an eligible way of earning money or privileges. At the very least, there should be alternative means available to such persons for obtaining the same benefits, lest the claim that the participation is voluntary be hollow indeed.[31]

I am, of course, assuming that subjecting oneself to hazardous medical experiments is different from many occupations that may involve similar levels of risk. This judgment is based not just on the circumstance that one is exposing one's body to permanent and perhaps subtle damage, with all this implies for one's sense of personal integrity, but also on the setting, the context in which this is done. A mountain climber may expose himself to risks, but he does so actively, by exercising his capacities to attain a goal that he can understand and attain. The experimental subject does not hazard his physical capacities by using them. Rather by abstracting his purposes from those in which his body is risked he makes his body into a separate thing which he sells or gives away, so that others may pursue *their* purposes with it.[32] It is only incidentally that the body so used belongs to a human being who has invested this body with his own personal identity and for whom it is the locus of purposes and integrity. To see the commercial traffic in human experimental subjects as simply another way of earning one's living is an extreme example of pressing certain kinds

---

[31] See Freund, "Introduction" to *Daedalus*.

[32] This general point is also made by Jonas, "Philosophical Reflections on Experimenting With Human Subjects" in *Daedalus*. For the philosophical discussion seeking to establish the connection between bodily and personal integrity, see Chapter 4.3.1.

of economic arguments into areas where they do not belong and past limits of which they do not take account.[33]

These considerations suggest the desirability of structuring experimentation so that the subject participates more fully than merely as an experimental animal. There is no problem, of course, if the experimentation is truly therapeutic — that is, if the search is for a cure for this patient's illness, and nothing is done that is not totally in the patient's interest. There is no problem, because the patient is not a subject at all, he is the object of personal care carried out with his health in mind. His body is no more being separated from the person as a whole than it is in standard treatment.

But where a subject is needed, the notion of participation suggests that those who are doing the intellectual work should also participate in the bodily labor — the risk, the pain, the waiting and discomfort. That some of the heroes of medical experimentation like Werner Forssman[34] and Daniel Carrion experimented first on themselves[35] is not a sign of these men's fanatic passion for

---

[33] This argument does not, I think, commit me to agreeing with Richard Titmuss's thesis in *The Gift Relationship — From Human Blood to Social Policy* (1971) that the commercial traffic in human blood is itself morally repellent. I feel the attractions of his position, but call attention to a significant difference. Although the passivity, the splitting off of body from person is present in both cases, in the case of blood the infringement is minimal, indeed insignificant, while in some cases of human experimentation the subject takes a major risk of being killed or maimed, or at least subjected to amounts of pain and discomfort which must interfere with his normal functioning.

[34] W. Forssmann, "The Role of Heart Catheterization and Angiocartography in the Development of Modern Medicine — Nobel Lecture (1956)" *Nobel Lectures, Physiology or Medicine, 1942–1962* (1964).

[35] Schultz, "Daniel Carrion's Experiment" 278 *N. Engl. J. Med.* 1323 (1968). Carrion, while an advanced medical student in the medical faculty in Lima at the end of the nineteenth century was concerned to study the incubation period and symptomatology of verruga peruana, a painful and frequently fatal disease afflicting primarily the Indian mountain dwellers of the Peruvian Andes. Believing that the disease was a Peruvian problem he felt it should be studied by a Peruvian, and as part of his studies deliberately inoculated himself with blood taken from a fourteen-year-old boy suffering from the disease. In less than two months he died as a result. It is said his experiments contributed significantly to the understanding of the disease. This and the previous references are excerpted in Katz.

knowledge, so much as it is a measure of their respect for fellow human beings, even those who might accept pay to be subjects. For had there been paid volunteers in Forssman's heart catheterization experiment, they surely would not have participated in his Nobel Prize. Indeed, the peculiar aptness of researchers treating themselves as subjects in the first instance is so striking that one wonders why this tradition has been so little appreciated.[36] Sometimes the researcher is not a fit subject; but where he is, can we not suppose that he feels it would be socially wasteful to expose *him* to risk, rather than a paid volunteer who could not make a corresponding intellectual contribution? This is, of course, just the kind of dehumanizing splitting of person and body that I am arguing against. If medicine advances somewhat more slowly, but the confidence of patients in the profession and the attitude of respect in the profession for the patient is maintained, I believe it will have been well worth it.

Certain therapies, however, can only be tested on persons suffering from the relevant disease, and unless the disease is to be artificially induced (if it can be), neither the researcher himself nor the very poor nor the institutionalized may represent a sufficient pool of subjects. What is to be done then? One perfectly possible strategy is to refrain from dangerous human experimentation except in cases where the experimental therapy is the only or the best chance for the individual in desperate cases, in the hope that sufficient data will be gathered eventually to bring the experimental therapy closer to the level of risk of the accepted alternative. Without doubt the general population would be the losers of such a strategy, in that better remedies would be more slowly developed and ineffective ones more slowly unmasked. But the price may be worth paying.

What is needed is a way out of this dilemma without preying on the disadvantage of vulnerable groups. Could we not call into play once more the notion of participation used in self-experimentation, but this time by making the class of beneficiaries, so far as possible,

---

[36] See generally Altman, "Auto-Experimentation — An Unappreciated Tradition in Medical Science" 286 *New Engl. J. Med.* 346 (February 17, 1972).

the same as the class put to risk by experiments? In this way each person would hazard his body in order to improve his health. One way of doing this, which I find unsatisfactory would have for instance the class of sufferers from Hodgkin's disease benefited by the experiments carried out on sufferers from Hodgkin's disease. Unfortunately, on closer inspection it appears that not all Hodgkin's disease sufferers will bear the cost of the experimentation from which all may benefit. What is even more troubling is the circumstance that it is those who are unfortunate enough to be sick who have to bear the burden not just of their illness but of the experimentation as well. Money compensation is at least a way of evening out *ex post* a serious inequity as to which any claim that *ex ante* we all had an equal chance of being stricken is a meaningless mockery.[37] But compensation has its own problems, as we have seen, certainly insofar as it is money compensation.

What, then, are we to do? The experts insist that experimentation and particularly clinical trials are crucial if medicine is to advance. Yet this does not mean that the advance is to be purchased by fraud or force or financial duress. Perhaps if the public were educated to the need for experimentation and to the often marginal nature of the sacrifices that the clinical trial asks — sacrifices that one should still be free to refuse — the public response might be entirely satisfactory.[38] The arguments against complete disclosure or for something of a forced draft for experimentation seem to me to express the experts' condescension towards the layman as much as a considered judgment as to what will or will not work. And, after all, if the public once fully informed refuses

---

[37] See Chapter 3.2.

[38] Richard Titmuss, in *The Gift Relationship* (1971), documents this assertion, at least in respect to blood donation. In Great Britain an entirely sufficient supply of blood is available for all purposes from voluntary donations. Although the propaganda for the blood donation program is low key, Titmuss shows that a sense of obligation, of gratitude and of community are adequate to assure that a large number of persons give blood regularly. The ethos of the National Health Service is likely to be a supporting factor in the maintenance of these attitudes. For criticism of some of Titmuss's theoretical analyses and conclusions, see Arrow, "Gifts and Exchanges" 1 *Philosophy and Public Affairs* 343 (1972) and the reply by Singer, "Altruism and Commerce" 2 *Philosophy and Public Affairs* 312 (1973).

to redefine its expectations of the profession to include the practice of experimentation, may this not be taken to show that progress is not that important to the consumers of medical care? And if it is not, who is to say they are wrong? I doubt whether we know that technical progress is as highly valued by the clientele of the profession as by the profession itself. Certainly secret or high-handed proceedings are no way to test that question, nor is relying on the paid participation of the poor and the captive.

What is needed first of all is candor and respect. This means that part of the energies of the profession should be devoted to educating the public in general, to educating individuals not only when they are sick and their participation is needed, but when they are well and thus not vulnerable. Then ways are needed of sharing the risks and benefits of experimentation, of clinical trials that demonstrably express the community between the sick and the healthy. If the participant in a clinical trial accepts special risks or gives up some of the security provided by the traditional concept of personal care, he would only participate freely if, when he was well, he saw himself as the beneficiary of similar sacrifices by others. Institutions must be devised to make palpable the bond of reciprocity between the sick and the well.[39] Whatever those institutions might look like, it seems quite clear that they cannot be exclusively governed by medical experts. Doctors and clients must decide together on what are useful and ethical experiments.

---

[39] These institutions might take many forms. Voluntary participation might be a single response on a single occasion by an individual whose help is needed. But greater formality might also be introduced. For instance a special medical plan might be offered to a large but limited pool of families. A very high level of care would be provided in return for the understanding that those in the pool would be asked to participate in clinical trials such as those summarized in the beginning of this chapter. The group would not be directed by doctors; rather the group would be self-ruled, with doctors and clients jointly deciding on the level of care to be provided and passing on the trials to be undertaken. Since the special care available would be costly, the outside world would have a great deal to say too about how valuable were the results of the research. Finally, although there would be an explicit moral obligation to do one's share once one's turn came, the obligation would not be legally enforceable and one could withdraw from the group at any time. In such a group the hazards of experimentation would be spread to the healthy as well as the ill, and compensation would be in a form that was related to the benefit provided.

Now we cannot be sure that greater candor, education and participation will resolve the dilemmas with which this essay has been concerned. None of the suggestions for accommodation in this final section can promise to do that. They do not promise a resolution, if by resolution is meant a scheme by which all the interests of society as a whole in having experimentation go forward are satisfied, while individual rights are respected. There is no reason to believe that such a resolution can necessarily be found. Rather it has been my more modest purpose to show how a more careful consideration of the system of rights may soften the dilemma and allow some experimentation to go forward. Indeed if anyone should offer a scheme by which the demands of efficiency could be met in full, it should properly be suspected that the proponent of such a scheme does not understand what rights are. It is the essence of rights to work as constraints on the pursuit of social goods. There is no guarantee that all will work out for the best, for this is not the best of all possible worlds.

A final word about money or other benefits, not as inducements for entering the experiment but as compensation for the harm that may be suffered. As matters stand, the situation is quite unsatisfactory. Chapter 2 sets out in detail how a paid volunteer is thought to have accepted and been paid for whatever risk eventuates, so that if things go wrong he has no special claim. And where the experimentation is in the course of treatment and no way is found to fault the treatment, once again there is no claim to compensation. But the argument of this section is that it is undesirable to rely on *ex ante* compensation to draw volunteers into experimentation, and that non-consensual experimentation in the course of treatment is just improper. Thus the theoretical argument supports the conclusions of Chapter 2 that schemes should be devised to offer *ex post* compensation to participants in medical experiments. I will not here repeat those conclusions or the discussion of the technical questions regarding the definition of harm, particularly where the experimentation is conducted in the course of treating sick subjects. It is sufficient to point out here how our willingness to offer such compensation serves the values developed in these

Chapters. *First*, it acknowledges that those who suffer harm in an experiment — if only because they received a nonstandard remedy that proved less effective than the standard — have done so in performing a service to others which under the ideal of personal care they were under no obligation to perform. The rest of us should now bear the cost. *Second*, it becomes possible to attract a category of subjects whose motives for participating are more in keeping with the ideal of participation, of joint venture discussed above. *Third*, if experimentation must bear the cost of the harm it does, there is some chance that it will be responsible and prudent and will be resorted to only when necessary.

Index